Praise for

SUFFERING SUCCOTASH

"Using humor, gusto, and her sensitive if skeptical palate to great effect, Stephanie Lucianovic explains the mechanics of picky eating. She shows us why we like some foods and not others, and illuminates the mysteries of our sense of taste. It takes a picky eater to understand picky eaters, and we should all be grateful for Lucianovic's inspired work."

—Amanda Hesser, cofounder of Food52.com and author of *The Essential New York Times Cookbook*

"As a diner who will gladly eat the eyeballs off a shrimp, but who recoils in horror at the sight of a raisin in an oatmeal cookie, I adored *Suffering Succotash*. Stephanie Lucianovic's charming and hilarious exploration of why we hate the foods we hate is packed to the gills with research on everything from sword-swallowers to supertasters and yet reads like a guilty pleasure. I couldn't put it down."

—Suzanne Morrison, author of *Yoga Bitch: One Woman's Quest to Conquer Skepticism, Cynicism, and Cigarettes on the Path to Enlightenment*

"Lucianovic proves that hanging out with a picky eater does not have to be torture—do not judge the picky eater, just laugh as she learns to enjoy cruciferous vegetables."

—Beth Lisick, author of *Helping Me Help Myself* and cocreator of Porchlight, the San Francisco storytelling series

"Hilarious and honest, *Suffering Succotash* is a fascinating read if you've ever gagged on your greens (or know someone who has)."

—Heather Cocks and Jessica Morgan, authors of *Spoiled* and cofounders of GoFugYourself.com

SUFFERING
SUCCOTASH

A Picky Eater's Quest to Understand
Why We Hate the Foods We Hate

Stephanie V.W. Lucianovic

A Perigee Book

A PERIGEE BOOK
Published by the Penguin Group
Penguin Group (USA) Inc.
375 Hudson Street, New York, New York 10014, USA
Penguin Group (Canada), 90 Eglinton Avenue East, Suite 700, Toronto, Ontario M4P 2Y3, Canada
(a division of Pearson Penguin Canada Inc.) • Penguin Books Ltd., 80 Strand, London WC2R 0RL,
England • Penguin Group Ireland, 25 St. Stephen's Green, Dublin 2, Ireland (a division of Penguin
Books Ltd.) • Penguin Group (Australia), 250 Camberwell Road, Camberwell, Victoria 3124, Australia
(a division of Pearson Australia Group Pty. Ltd.) • Penguin Books India Pvt. Ltd., 11 Community
Centre, Panchsheel Park, New Delhi—110 017, India • Penguin Group (NZ), 67 Apollo Drive,
Rosedale, Auckland 0632, New Zealand (a division of Pearson New Zealand Ltd.) • Penguin Books
(South Africa) (Pty.) Ltd., 24 Sturdee Avenue, Rosebank, Johannesburg 2196, South Africa
Penguin Books Ltd., Registered Offices: 80 Strand, London WC2R 0RL, England

While the author has made every effort to provide accurate telephone numbers, Internet
addresses, and other contact information at the time of publication, neither the publisher nor the
author assumes any responsibility for errors, or for changes that occur after publication. Further,
the publisher does not have any control over and does not assume any responsibility
for author or third-party websites or their content.

First edition: July 2012

Library of Congress Cataloging-in-Publication Data

Lucianovic, Stephanie V. W.
Suffering succotash : a picky eater's quest to understand why we hate the foods
we hate / Stephanie V.W. Lucianovic.— 1st ed.
p. cm.
ISBN 978-0-399-53750-9 (pbk.)
1. Senses and sensation—Popular works. 2. Taste buds—Popular works. 3. Food preferences—
Popular works. 4. Nutrition—Psychological aspects—Popular works. I. Title.
QP431.L83   2012
612.8084'6—dc23   2012008772

PRINTED IN THE UNITED STATES OF AMERICA

10 9 8 7 6 5 4 3 2 1

PUBLISHER'S NOTE: Neither the publisher nor the author is engaged in rendering professional
advice or services to the individual reader. The ideas, procedures, and suggestions contained in this
book are not intended as a substitute for consulting with your physician. All matters regarding your
health require medical supervision. Neither the author nor the publisher shall be liable or responsible
for any loss or damage allegedly arising from any information or suggestion in this book.

The recipes contained in this book are to be followed exactly as written. The publisher is
not responsible for your specific health or allergy needs that may require medical supervision.
The publisher is not responsible for any adverse reactions to the recipes contained in this book.

Some names and identifying characteristics have been changed to
protect the privacy of the individuals involved.

Most Perigee books are available at special quantity discounts for bulk purchases for
sales promotions, premiums, fund-raising, or educational use. Special books, or book
excerpts, can also be created to fit specific needs. For details, write: Special Markets,
Penguin Group (USA) Inc., 375 Hudson Street, New York, New York 10014.

To my family, including the members with tails,
for all their love, patience, and laughs.

CONTENTS

Three More Bites and You're Done

For years I've pondered the question of what exactly made me so hate so many foods for so long. Was it the texture, color, or odor of the foods, or just a primal need to fight the parental power of enforced eating? Eh, I couldn't tell you. I just knew I dreaded most mealtimes, and my older sister, Jennie, was just as picky.

Three years older, wiser, and stronger, Jennie broke most of the boundaries parents set out for children to break, and I followed (or not) as I saw fit. The truth is, I was fairly chicken about the whole boundary-breaking thing, and I really just wanted to avoid getting into trouble. Yet . . . I wanted to avoid food even more, so in those cases, where Jennie led, I followed. At a safe distance.

Even with my parents' fairly generous "Three Bites Rule," Jennie and I were determined never to eat more of any food we hated than strictly necessary. If we were really crafty, we wouldn't even have to *taste* a molecule of the food we were avoiding. After years of careful research and development, we designed a highly complex system of food avoidance techniques.

My parents' way of getting food into us without making the actual act of eating a punishment was to use the Three Bites Rule. As in, "Three more bites and you never have to see that particular serving of succotash again."

As devised by my parents (hereafter referred to as "The Enforcers"), the Three Bites Rule (hereafter referred to as "The Rule") was understood by the children (hereafter referred to as "The Picky Eaters") to be the following:

1. The Picky Eaters shall not invoke the The Rule at the beginning of the meal, as some part of the full helping must be ingested before requesting the application of The Rule.
2. For a bite to be counted and therefore subtracted from the overall tally, The Picky Eaters must be observed ingesting the bite by The Enforcers of The Rule.
3. An "acceptable" bite is required to be of sufficient volume. Said volume will be determined by The Enforcers of The Rule. For instance, a "bite" is not any of the following: a pea, a 1-millimeter piece of meat, half of a scalloped potato round, or a grain of wild rice.

We accepted The Rule as stated, but we still did everything we could to avoid eating any part of a hated helping of food. For that, Jennie and I contrived loopholes circumventing The Rule.

Loophole 1. Apply the "Push and Hide" maneuver. Push small portions of the Despised Food around the plate to give the appearance of disturbance that occurs naturally when eating. While in the process of pushing, take the opportunity to secrete some of the Despised Food in other places. Detritus such as gnawed bones or discarded potato skins, for instance, provide good coverage for this particular act. Because of the dispersal, the "Push and Hide" method has the added effect of making it appear as though there is less Despised Food on the plate.

Loophole 2. Follow the "Pantomime Procedure." Load a fork with an adequate mouthful of the Despised Food and raise it to the mouth, but do not ingest. Quickly lower the still-full fork to the plate and go through chewing motions. Take special care not to bite the inside of the cheek, which would result in a loud yelp, calling attention to the fact that the mouth is actually empty. In the event of being observed while the fork is en route to the mouth, fall back to the "Don't Talk with Your Mouth Full" position.

Loophole 3. Assume the "Don't Talk with Your Mouth Full" position. Because it follows that, when talking, one should lower the full fork to the plate to avoid the accusation of bad manners, say the first thing that comes to mind if observed with a full fork positioned at, but not entering, the mouth. However, be aware that saying the first thing that comes to mind might have unforeseen and potentially detrimental ramifications. Consider whether making "I tipped Mr. Leebens's jar of pancreas upside down and got formaldehyde all over me," or "I'm not staying after school for yearbook because I got detention for setting the chem lab on fire" known to the general public is an acceptable price to pay to avoid the Despised Food.

No matter when applied, the Three Bites Rule was pretty much always accompanied by loud—but not completely staged—gagging as we gulped cheekfuls of water to wash down each bite like medication. That way we didn't have to chew anything, and if we didn't have to chew anything, we didn't have to taste anything. If you chewed and *then* gulped, you were doing it wrong.

The Gulp and Swallow Method

Best Way
1. Fill mouth with water.
2. Carefully insert first bite.
3. Swallow all.
4. Repeat with bites two and three.

However, the above is admittedly difficult as you run the risk of spewing water across the table. While it involves one more step and potentially tasting the Despised Food, it is much safer and less damp to forgo the initial mouthful of water with the Easier Way:

Easier Way
1. Pinch nose to minimize impact of food on taste buds.
2. Carefully insert first bite at back of tongue to minimize impact of food on taste buds.
3. Chug water and swallow all.
4. Repeat with bites two and three.

My dad really hated this practice, because even though

we were technically following the Three Bites Rule to the letter, he suspected we were getting away with something. Since he couldn't say exactly *what* we were getting away with, he instead took solace in lecturing that we weren't getting any nutritional value this way and, therefore, we shouldn't be allowed to do it. Number one, kids don't care about nutrition, so using that as an argument isn't going to get you anywhere. (More to the point, kids will happily eat anything if they're assured that it has no nutritional value whatsoever. I even boycotted orange popsicles because I was convinced it was my mother's way of tricking me into eating something that was good for me.) Number two, it's false. As I've come to learn in my adulthood, as long as the food hits your stomach, chewed up or not, it's going to get absorbed into your bloodstream. How else do you explain oysters?

Even with all the loopholes and the two branches of Gulp and Swallow, there were still times when even the Three Bites Rule was too much for us, and as such, we concocted some elaborate and spectacularly faulty schemes for dispatching our food without ever actually putting it in our mouths: the "Pets as Trash Compactors Gambit," the "Baked Potato Skin Contingency Plan," and "Retch Softly and Carry a Large Napkin." I think you get my point: picky.

While I dreaded most mealtimes as a picky kid, at least I had an action plan back then. As a picky adult, it wasn't quite so easy, because not only did I have a feeling my friends wouldn't appreciate my throwing food at their pets during dinner parties, but most people think of picky eating as a kid thing, so I sort of knew that I was expected to have grown out of the picky stage. As a college student, I was expected to go out to fancy dinners with boyfriends' parents and enthusiastically partake of the smoked whipped fish they'd ordered for the table. (And I was supposed to do it without retching, if you can believe that.) Later, as a young urban professional, I was expected to agree enthusiastically to dim sum brunches in Boston's Chinatown without revealing how much I was freaking out about what exactly was hiding in those little dumplings.

At that time, being a picky eater was so much a part of who I was and had always been that I never questioned the whys and wherefores of it. The way I figured it, some people like vegetables and fish the same way some people's favorite color is brown. It's clearly bizarre and totally against the laws of nature, but it's the way things are, and there's just no explaining it. But then I started to become *un*picky. I started cooking more than frozen foods; I watched the Food Network and subscribed to every glossy food magazine the newsstands had to offer. I started to really enjoy a lot of food. Then I took it a few steps further and went to culinary school, started a food blog, became a food writer and editor, and before you could say "bon appétit," I was a full-blown foodie annoying the diners around me by taking dark and blurry photos of every single meal I ate out.

Enjoying food wasn't a first for me. I'd always enjoyed stuffing out on the foods I really liked, but things got weird when I started to love the foods I'd once hated and avoided with all my might. Because, like, what the hell just happened? One minute, I'm agreeing with the entire pop culture universe that Brussels sprouts are the grossest thing in the world, and the next I'm buying pounds of them at farmers' markets and ordering them in restaurants. Did I finally just grow up, or are they now genetically modifying vegetables to be less grody? I had to get to the bottom of this weird metamorphosis in case I suddenly woke up craving bugs or something.

One potential explanation I kept coming across was that as you age, your taste buds die out; therefore, when you're a kid, everything tastes so much stronger than as an adult. Okay, so that might explain why I now like Brussels sprouts, but it doesn't explain why I still hate the texture of rice pudding. The R.I.P. Taste Buds theory also doesn't explain why some kids out there (like my husband) never go through a picky phase, so there must be other explanations.

What I didn't expect to find were answers to questions I hadn't even thought to ask, like the badass and very scientific explanation why some picky eaters don't like their foods to touch. And what a flower show smackdown in 1935 has to do with the way we taste things as individuals. Did I need to go into deep therapy to discover that my original pickiness really stemmed from a bratty need to thwart my parents? And maybe I was about to discover that, because I can pinpoint my first flashes of depickification to our first dates, maybe my husband (the human garbage disposal) has actually been brainwashing me all these years! And ultimately, if I could figure out what made me a picky eater, could I also pinpoint what caused it in others?—something that, as a new mom, was causing me not a little bit of anxiety.

What nonpicky eaters don't seem to grasp is that picky eaters don't choose to be picky. Picky eaters don't even like the word "picky." (Or for that matter, "finicky," "fussy," or "persnickety," all of which describe a personality trait, not a diet choice. Are there better words out there to describe our, uh, condition? Well, some of the more technical or medical terms I've heard are "selective eating," or "severe food refusal," neither of which is any easier to digest than "picky" or "finicky.") Vocabulary building aside, ask any picky eater you know whether, if given the choice, they'd stay picky. Some may say that they've long accepted their pickiness and shrug off any potential to change, but others would leap at the opportunity to eat more foods. Some picky eaters, myself included, have been able to get past a lot of their picky predilections. Others simply can't. Not won't, *can't*. But why can't they? And why could I? Vegans and vegetarians get to have a cause to fall back on and deliver stinging lectures on the evils of animal products. But where's our cause? We don't really have one. Picky eaters just get eye rolls, and our only defense or attempt at an explanation generally runs along the lines of, "Yeah, well, I don't eat raisins because I don't *like* raisins!" That's not effective. There's got to be a better way to explain why picky eaters are the way they are (and why raisins are so damn disgusting).

It is high time someone got to the bottom of this, and given how long I studied the craft of picky eating as an amateur, it might as well be me. So while everyone else is writing books like *What I Ate for Love*, or *My Year with Funyons* (followed by its sequel, *My Year Without Funyons*), or *I Can't Believe I Ate the Whole Farm! (But I Did and Now I'm Going to Tell You All About It)*, I'm writing about what we *don't* eat. I'm writing about what makes us gag. I'm writing about the foods we hate, disdain, despise, and otherwise plain don't get along with, and trying to find out exactly *why* we feel that way—and why sometimes we don't anymore.

It just occurred to me that by fully explicating how my sister and I brilliantly eluded the three-bites-and-you're-done rule, I just gave my son a handbook on how to avoid food at my dinner table. Oh, well, picky eating's not hereditary. Or is it?

CHAPTER 1

Blame the Supertaster

The human tongue is not meant to be examined up close. The bumps on my tongue look gross, a bunch of skin tags hanging out over the edges of a hole punched in a piece of stiff paper. Staring intently into a mirror clouded by my son's smudgy fingerprints, I am getting up close and personal with my papillae, which are currently an intense and extremely unhealthy shade of blue.

According to a how-to I found online, swabbing some blue food coloring on your tongue will indeed turn it blue, but your papillae (the bumps on your tongue where your taste buds live) are supposed to stay pink, making them easier to count. Clearly, I don't know what "some" means because, gauging by my reflection, absolutely every possible surface on my tongue has turned a deep, dark blue, making me look more like a strangled corpse in an Agatha Christie movie than someone performing a scientific experiment. I see no easy-to-count pink papillae, the number of which is so crucial to finding out if I can blame my picky eating on being a supertaster.

Currently, picky eating is destined to go down as one of life's great mysteries, because it's fantastically hard to pinpoint the cause. It could be in your genes, it could be a psychological issue, it could be your parents' fault for making you clean your plate, or it could be all those things smashed together with a bunch of other factors. One idea that has gotten lots of recent media attention is that picky eaters are frequently part of an elite group known as supertasters.

When I first heard the term "supertaster" being bandied about the foodie and food blogger world a few years ago, I assumed that being one meant your tongue could do what Geordi's visor did in *Star Trek: The Next Generation*: provide a comprehensive and detailed analysis of anything in its range, no matter how complex or varied. Sadly it's nothing so grand or cool. Very simply, supertasters are people who are genetically predisposed to be highly sensitive to certain foods (coffee, grapefruit, Brussels sprouts, and broccoli are a few examples) that have flavor profiles similar to the chemical propylthiouracil (PROP), a bitter compound found in some plants.

This means that *if* I'm a supertaster, it's not my fault! It's my genetics that made me refuse those horrid damp piles of string beans, peas, succotash, and spinach for so many years. "Don't look at me, Mom and Dad—they're *your* genes!" Ah, justice, it would be sweet.

However, a lot of articles—including an online supertaster test on the BBC website—make the leap that being sensitive to those flavors automatically translates into active dislike. Right there, that puts a stopper in blaming my genetics for my picky past, because I actually really *like* grapefruit, Brussels sprouts, coffee, broccoli, and cabbage. Not only that, but I seek out the bitterest beers I can find—the hoppier they are, the happier I am. My bitter obsession makes me wonder if I could possibly be what the science community calls an "undertaster," which sounds like my tongue is a slack-ass underachiever that is bound to be a constant source of disappointment to me.

The polar opposite of supertasters, undertasters are taste insensitive to bitter flavors. Undertasters—sometimes dubbed "taste-blind"—can't detect the existence of PROP. Therefore, they are less likely to be put off by any taste of bitterness in foods, and as a result, they are less likely to be picky eaters. Dr. Mehmet Oz's book *You on a Diet* states that 25% of the population are supertasters, 50% are average tasters, and the remaining 25% are undertasters.

Confused about where being a recovering picky eater who now likes bitter foods leaves me and the tongue I hope to scapegoat, I contacted my first taste expert. Professor Virginia Utermohlen of Cornell University's Taste Science Laboratory helped develop the BBC's online supertaster test, and since academic departments make researchers' and stalkers' lives easier by listing everyone's email addresses right on their websites, I am able to fire off a carefully written email directly to Professor Utermohlen asking if she has the time to answer some questions about supertasters and picky eating. Less than three hours later, I get Professor Utermohlen's warm and welcoming response: "Sure! What questions do you have?"

What follows is a thrilling night of back-and-forth emails during which Professor Utermohlen sets quite a few things straight. First off, the good professor actually prefers the term "highly sensitive tasters" to "supertaster." As she explains, "[Supertaster] isn't an accurate term, and I don't think there is anything particularly 'super' about being a supertaster." Given that so many supertasters seem to end up suffering as picky eaters, I agree with her there. Professor Utermohlen then goes on to dispel the anecdotal idea that there are specific foods supertasters universally dislike: "It's more that highly sensitive tasters have foods they dislike intensely, but the actual food varies from person to person." Furthermore, being extra-sensitive to certain flavors doesn't necessarily mean you dislike those flavors. "For example," Dr. Utermohlen writes, "I am just now telling myself not to eat any more of the wonderfully 'bitter' chocolate I have next to me (eighty-six percent cacao . . .), but I hate beer and Brussels sprouts, and find grapefruit far too bitter." There you have it: My fondness for bitter beer, coffee, and other bitter foods has little to no bearing on my potential supertastiness.

A quick Internet search unearths a handful of ways to determine if you're a supertaster. All the tests appear to be geared toward determining if the test taker is unusually sensitive to bitterness. Two of them are actual taste tests that involve how strongly a bitter compound tastes, and the other makes you go cross-eyed counting your tongue bumps to see if you have the required number to be taste sensitive. Some can be executed with a minimal amount of fuss and expense, and others require very deep pockets or knowing the right geneticist. Since I am not currently sitting on pots of gold, I decide to give the at-home, budget-friendly tests a go.

The Sweet'N Low Test

Dr. Mehmet Oz—the eminent cardiothoracic surgeon, whom you might also know as "Oprah's Dr. Oz" if you watch the amount of TV I do—wrote on Esquire.com about a quick and dirty taste test you can do at home to determine your supertastiness.

His directions are as follows:

> Mix a packet of Sweet'N Low into half a glass of water and put a spoonful on your tongue. If you taste bitter, you're a supertaster. If you taste sweet, you're an undertaster. (If you taste both, you don't need to be reading this.)

Lest you be under some misapprehension that I'm a chill, laid-back sort of gal, let me explain why this test pisses me off with its inattention to desperately important minutiae.

Instantly, my detail-oriented cook's brain goes crazy over the "half a glass of water" directive. What size glass? Does he mean "half a cup"? My pint glasses and POM Wonderful souvenir glasses are both 16 ounces (yes, I measured), so are we talking 8 ounces? Or by "glass," does he mean a juice glass and that half of that would be 4 ounces? Come on, man, my foodie cred and picky eating past are at stake here; I am *not* messing around!

Ultimately, I go with the 16/8-ounce measurement and mix in a packet of Sweet'N Low generously and unknowingly provided by the Stanford Math Department. I ladle the liquid onto my tongue, hold it there, and exert masterful control over my impulse to swallow the grody mixture. I concentrate hard on my tongue. Yes, I taste sweetness, but there is some bitterness, too. When I spit the solution out, I definitely taste residual bitterness. In the interest of completeness, I perform the test a few more times to be sure and get the same result: I taste both bitter and sweet.

> *Sweet'N Low Test Result:* **DON'T NEED TO BE READING THIS.**

The Blue Tongue Test

People show and tell you strange things when they find out you're writing a book. During a play date, I happen to mention my blue tongue experiment to a friend, which prompts her to respond with the news that her son's allergist thinks she might have "geographic tongue." Then she opens her mouth wide and proceeds to show me what she's talking about. I've heard that this sort of thing happens to doctors all the time, but I didn't expect it to happen because I was writing a book about picky eating.

You really want to scare yourself? Do an Internet image search for "geographic tongue," and you'll be inundated with a bunch of tongues that look segmented or deeply creased in parts. Other tongues sport what look like bald patches. The condition comes about when the tongue's papillae die off in a certain area. According to the Mayo Clinic, geographic tongue, which is harmless, got its name because when one patch of denuded papillae heals, the condition moves to another part of the tongue. It's the tongue equivalent of continental drift. And because I can't leave well enough alone, I follow the Mayo Clinic's link to a related condition known as "black, hairy tongue." Resulting from an excess of bacteria, black, hairy tongue—which seems to be its official name, it doesn't even get a technical nom de plume in the way that geographic tongue is also called "benign migratory glossitis"— has the unfortunate effect of giving your tongue a very fine toupee. The Mayo Clinic notes, "Although black, hairy tongue may look alarming, it doesn't cause any health problems." (*May?!*) It might comfort some to know that black, hairy tongue usually goes away without needing medical intervention. Not me. If my tongue suddenly started asking for its own razor, and there was nothing any doctor could do about it, I'd think seriously about rinsing my mouth out with Nair. And that's where I stop myself from looking up all the other tongue conditions listed on the Mayo Clinic's addictive website and prep for my second at-home, budget-friendly supertaster test.

My first order of business is to answer a questionnaire on the BBC website that is paired with their version of the Blue Tongue Test. The questionnaire offers an invitation to "[f]ind out whether you live in the intense world of a supertaster or whether most foods you eat taste pretty much the same" and then administers a personality test in order to diagnose taster status. For example, one of the questions is, "You are planning to go to a fine restaurant with friends. Which restaurant would you prefer?" and the choices are, "A small, quiet, cosy restaurant with simple décor," "An elegant restaurant with mirrors and an outdoor patio," and "A popular busy restaurant with a large dining room where you can see everything that's going on." Another question asks, "15 minutes later, the food has just arrived. Do you . . ." "Tuck in straight away without really thinking about it," "Taste a small mouthful and try to distinguish the different flavours," or "Take in the food's aroma—the food has to smell good for you to really enjoy eating it."

You get the idea. There are five questions, and at the end, the answers determine the number of papillae on the test taker's tongue. For the record, my answers jibe with my Sweet'N Low Test and relegate me to the "normal taster" category. (Remember, 50% of the population is that boring. *Sigh*.)

"Whatever," I grumble to myself, laying out the materials needed for the Blue Tongue Test next to the bathroom sink. "Like I'm going to believe some Q and A that sounds like things foodies would ask on a speed date."

Slightly higher-tech than the two-ingredient Sweet'N Low Test I subjected myself to earlier, the BBC's Blue Tongue Test requires cotton swabs, blue food coloring, a magnifying glass, and reinforcement rings. If you're like me and stopped stocking reinforcement rings around the time you stopped lugging around a kitten-plastered Trapper Keeper, an index card punched with a 7mm hole punch will do just as well.

And that's how I have come to be in my bathroom dealing with the fact that my incredibly unattractive papillae have not remained the required pink, which means that either I have oversaturated them with food coloring or they simply don't want to stand up and be counted. After striking a few truly sad attempts at Gene Simmons poses, I resalivate and swallow a couple of times and finally manage to dilute the blue dye enough to see my swollen pink papillae shining up among the rest of the blue tongue flesh.

Next, I stick the hole-punched index card on the front of my tongue and lean across the bathroom vanity, smack up against the mirror. Right around the time I start to go blind in my attempt to count the tiny shiny dots—pink they may be, but tiny they still are—I pull out a small plastic magnifying glass, but I can't wrangle the right angle to see all the papillae in their magnified state. The longer I fuss, the harder it gets, because my mouth breathing is now starting to fog up both the mirror and the magnifier.

With the hole-punched index card still plastered against my tongue, I summon my husband, gesturing with the magnifier that I need his help in counting. Of course, he tries to ask me a lot of questions, which, since my tongue is hanging out the entire time, only elicit slightly guttural, dentist-hand-in-mouth responses from me.

Mark: Should I count the rows of bumps or go from the outside in, counting in concentric circles?

Mark: If half a bump is half under the paper edge and half exposed, is it counted or not?

Mark: Can you make your tongue drier? Your saliva is making it hard to see the bumps clearly.

Mark: You know, I really should put the paper hole over several different areas of your tongue to get an accurate count. Don't you think that's a good idea?

Mark: Your face is turning red. Is that a side effect of the food coloring?

After a couple of attempts at repositioning the magnifier and trying to count my papillae from new angles and distances, Mark announces he's going to get the digital camera. I flap my arms and gabble incoherently, clearly indicating that while I vastly appreciate his precision, dedication, and the great lengths to which he is willing to go to facilitate my experiment, and that while I will remain indebted to him for allowing me to trespass on his working hours, I really feel there is no need to document the procedure with photographic evidence.

Pretending not to understand anything I just grunted, Mark proceeds to take twenty-four photos of my tongue in various lights and then gets irritated when I am unable to sit still for the extreme close-ups. At one point, he switches off all the lights and shines a flashlight down on my tongue to illuminate the subject. While we look at the resulting photos on my computer, Mark makes some comment about my bulging papillae looking like a Georgia O'Keeffe painting. I tell him if that's a Georgia O'Keeffe, someone better smear the canvas with Valtrex.

In the end, Mark is convinced I have 30 papillae in the 7mm area, whereas I counted only 25. The BBC site says at least 35 papillae are needed to be a supertaster; however, other sources say 20 to 25 earn you the title.[1]

Blue Tongue Test Result: INCONCLUSIVE.

This clearly hazy area of exactly how many papillae it takes to make a supertaster gives me another glimmer of

---

1. Oh, Internet-based research, how I love your vagueness.

hope that I'm not just an average taster. That hope is further bolstered when Dr. Utermohlen notes that it's not necessarily about the quantity of papillae, it's more about how sensitive each of them is. You could have scads of papillae, but if the nerve endings aren't sensitive enough, you won't be a supertaster. On the other hand, you might have an average number of papillae, but if each of them houses very sensitive taste buds, that would make you more taste sensitive than someone with an obscene mass of papillae containing less sensitive taste buds.

The Taste Test

With my tongue still singing the blues, I move on to the next step in my self-experimentation by scoring a chemistry kit of taste tests from an online science lab supply store. Can you believe a lab supply store allows run-of-the-mill people to buy this kind of stuff? If you're interested in outfitting your dungeon laboratory (which must be pronounced "la-bora-tory," followed by an evil laugh), other things you can buy include materials to build electrodes, glass Erlenmeyer flasks (those are the triangular bottles mad scientists are always drinking from), and my favorite, the glass burettes.

Burettes are long, thin glass tubes that are filled with liquids and clamped into a stand. Using a tiny valve called a stopcock at one end of the burette, the liquid flow can be switched on and off, allowing for the measurement of very minute amounts of the liquid. With a touch of the stopcock, you can dispense liquid in a continuous stream or slow it down to drop by drop.

I'm now trying to find a culinary reason why a burette is essential to my kitchen.

The taste test kit consists of 100 each of sodium benzoate test strips, thiourea test strips, and PTC (phenylthiocarbamide/phenylthiourea) taste test strips. A bitter compound, PTC is chemically similar to PROP and both are used—along with sodium benzoate and thiourea—in taste perception tests. Also included in my little chemistry kit is the item that solidifies this as a true science experiment: the control test strips. Awesome.[2]

I am momentarily flummoxed to discover that the very scientific-looking plastic vials of test strips arrive with zero instructions. Not that it's, uh, rocket science or anything, but I wonder if I need to prep my mouth in some way. Rinse it? Use one of those tongue scrapers? Stop drinking this cup of tepid coffee? Also, do I need to follow a progression of taste tests, like in cheese tasting, where you go from mildest to stinkiest, so you don't blow out all your taste buds in the first mouthful? (See? Obsessed with precision.)

The brightly colored slips of paper in each vial do have directions but they are of a different sort. The control paper vial announces, "THIS PAPER IS INERT AND TASTELESS." The thiourea and sodium benzoate vials holler, "KEEP WELL-STOPPERED AND AWAY FROM LIGHT." Finally, the PTC

---

2. Even more awesome is that the excessive number of strips means I have plenty to spare. It means that after I test myself, I can taste-test everyone around. Parents, sisters, friends, son, husband—no one will be safe from my bitter little strips. "Are you a supertaster? Boom! Just proved it!" I might even start taste-testing strangers on the street just for the hell of it. Then again, asking Northern Californians to stick a piece of paper on their tongue that *doesn't* give them an acid trip might be slightly dangerous.

vial warns, "Each individual should take the taste test only once." Next to the screaming caps on the other papers, this most alarming note comes across as oddly subdued in its lowercase type. You'd think that would be the note they'd want capped, boldfaced, and wrapped in yellow police tape. (I would learn later that PTC is a potent thyroid toxin, so that's why you wouldn't want to keep sucking on papers coated with it.)

My brain reaches back to what I once knew about science experiments from high school and recalls that the whole point of a control is to correct for nothing because even nothing can do something, and it's important to know what it does. Or doesn't do. Since I am not conducting a blind taste test on myself and there is nothing on the "inert" control strip, there is probably no reason to taste it. But just in case the nothing turns out to be something—and also to stop this train of thought from pushing me through the looking glass—I decide to taste something of the nothingness. After rolling the strip of paper on my tongue for a good thirty seconds, I can definitely confirm something: Nothing is there.

Although the vials themselves don't have anything telling me how to conduct the taste tests, the site I bought them from does have some procedural instructions, which are pretty simple and basically along the lines of, "Put paper on tongue. Taste it." The three possible results for the PTC test are, "no response; slight bitter taste; revolting." ("Revolting" is a highly scientific term.)

Accepting the fact that I might be about to voluntarily taste something "revolting," I take a deep breath and start tasting the other strips. Oh, who am I kidding? I am *hoping* I'll taste something revolting and not just because it might mean I'm a supertaster, but because deep down, I am still a kid who wants to push the gross-out limits. You can then imagine how disappointed I end up being with my tragically boring results. Given that I can taste stuff on the strips but nothing actually revolts me, it appears I am still in "average taster" territory and getting tired of both the ambiguity and the mediocrity. To liven the experiment up, I pull Mark out of his office for a truly blind taste test.

He proceeds to taste absolutely nothing on every strip, accuses me of giving him four control test trips, informs me that "experimenting on yourself is generally considered to be unethical," and then gets really annoyed when he learns that one of the tasteless-to-him strips was sodium benzoate. (Mark carries a grudge against sodium benzoate because the cat repellent we use to keep our cats from tipping over the study trashcan has sodium benzoate in it. Every time Mark touches his trashcan without thinking, he gets the extremely bitter repellent all over his hands and somehow manages to then get it in his mouth.) Mark insists on testing another sodium benzoate strip, and since it doesn't carry the disturbing "once is enough, my friend" warning that the PTC strips do, I let him. Not content to let half the strip hang out of his mouth, he shoves the whole strip in and chews it for maximum effect. Still nothing. Although our son has yet to exhibit taster signs in any way, it already looks like Mark's tongue is the underachiever in this house. No wonder he's never had a picky moment in his life. It also explains why he eats everything I cook. (And I mean everything. Even when I thought baking avocado onto a pizza was a good idea.)

My Results
PTC: slightly bitter
Sodium benzoate: kind of sour, slightly sulfurous
Thiourea: slightly bitter
Control: nothing

My Taste Test Result: AVERAGE TASTER

Mark's Results
PTC: nothing
Sodium benzoate: nothing
Thiourea: nothing
Control: nothing

Mark's Taste Test Result: AVERAGE TASTER

Henry's Results
Mark won't let me experiment on our thirteen-month-
   old son.

Since we get the taster genes from our parents, I test my
parents during one of their visits to the West Coast and record
the results. My mother has pretty much the same reactions
I did. My dad, however:

PTC: "Tastes like paper."
Sodium benzoate: "Tastes like paper."
Thiourea: "Tastes like paper."
Control: "Tastes like paper."

Like Mark, it looks like Dad's an undertaster, although he

thinks the extreme allergies he's had all his life might have messed up his sense of smell and taste. Whatever the reason, for the rest of the weekend, he uses it as an excuse to eat double—sometimes triple—helpings of everything. "Might as well have all of it; can't taste anything anyway," he says in aggrieved tones and then adds, "See, that's why I have to eat so much food—it's the only way I'll taste it."

"No, Vern," my mom counters, "you just have a tapeworm."

As exciting it was to get the mad scientist package in the mail, this test ends personally anticlimactic. I was really hoping to have a near-vomiting reaction or, at the very least, a good, hard gag. Frankly, I was looking to have the reaction my friend Rachel had when I taste-tested her several weeks later. After allowing the PTC strip to briefly touch her tongue, Rachel, who doesn't drink much, actually pours herself a new glass of wine in order to wash the PTC taste out of her mouth, exclaiming, "Ew, *ew*! That's horribly bitter! Why did you do that to me? I gotta eat something!" She splashes out more rosé and tells me—between desperate pink gulps—that the PTC tastes like bile rising out of her throat. She is clearly revolted, just as the PTC instructions predicted.

Throughout these tests, I keep reminding myself that Dr. Utermohlen said that taste sensitivity is not easy to measure. The only way to prove beyond a shadow of a doubt that I am (or am not) a supertaster is to call in the big guns.

The Genetic Test

At long last, it is time to dig up some geneticists. The DIY tests are all well and good, but getting your genes analyzed to determine their taster status (also known as their genotype) is the only conclusive, scientific proof whether or not someone is a supertaster.

When I start looking into how I could prevail upon some willing geneticist to take time out of their busy day deciphering the human genome to attend to my personal quest, I discover that you can buy almost anything on the Internet these days. Including your genetic analysis.

23andMe.com, a genetic testing site (tagline: "Genetics just got personal," which, I'm sorry, sounds like something out of a movie trailer), charges $399–$499 to genotype you. If you dig deep into your pockets and go this route, 23andMe sends you a mailable saliva kit (with the postage prepaid to avoid uncomfortable questions from the postal worker in charge of weighing your package of bodily fluids[3]), and once you send back your carefully harvested spit, your genetic analysis will be made available to you in a secure online form.

While the idea of sending my saliva through the mail to be analyzed does make me feel wonderfully dramatic and a bit like a soap opera character trying to determine if it was really her brother that she slept with while dealing with the amnesia she got when her evil twin threw her down a well, my wallet runs more to the "buy blue food coloring, but steal Sweet'N Low from a university break room" category, as it did for my other tests. I decide to back-burner 23andMe for now and see if I can track down a geneticist who would be willing to help a poor writer out for a cut rate.

---

3. It's legal to send bodily fluids through the USPS? Who knew?

My search for a sympathetic geneticist and my desire to compose a halfway intelligent, nongibbering email has me looking up unpronounceable words such as "dysgeusia," the term used when the sense of taste becomes distorted.[4] Dysgeusia is one of a family of taste terms: "Hypogeusia" occurs if your sense of taste is decreased, and "ageusia" is when you lose your sense of taste completely, which is what happened to my grandfather after he banged his head falling off a coal train at the General Motors factory. The search also has me asking my husband, "Do PhDs prefer to be addressed as 'doctor' or 'professor'? Which one would flatter them more so they would be more likely to talk to me?"

Dr. Danielle Reed, who is a Member[5] of Monell Chemical Senses Center—an independent, nonprofit scientific institute in Philadelphia, whose research focuses exclusively on studying the senses of taste and smell—is the geneticist who kindly responds to my plea and tells me they'll send me a cheek-swabbing kit with instructions. When I get her email, I am so geeked out that I actually squeal most unscientifically.

Monell's media office also sends reading material on PTC/PROP, picky eating, and the very important TAS2r38 gene. When this passel of fairly heavy reading material hits my in-box, I settle down to decipher the science jargon with a red pen and a dictionary.

---

4. My mother will be so proud. If none of her daughters became scientists, at least one of them is writing like one. Sort of.

5. When I asked what her title was, Dr. Reed responded with an email that had the subject line: "Title=Queen<joke>." Scientists are hysterical! Dr. Reed then explained that "Member" at Monell is like being a professor at other universities.

Just for a refresher, aside from our bitter old friend, the human tongue can detect four other tastes: sweet, sour, salty, and umami. If you aren't familiar with that last one, don't blame yourself. Umami, which is best described as the taste of "savoriness" and found in meats, cheeses, and mushrooms, was discovered only about a hundred years ago by a Japanese chemist.

According to the Umami Information Center, Dr. Kikunae Ikeda of Tokyo University was analyzing dashi (the seaweed broth used in miso soup, among other Japanese dishes) in order to "ascertain the true nature of [its] 'deliciousness.'" (I want a job where I determine the true nature of the deliciousness of foods. That would definitely make a burette necessary, don't you think?) Dr. Ikeda decided that dashi's deliciousness sprung from the seaweed's main active ingredient: glutamate (or glutamic acid).[6] In 1912, Dr. Ikeda addressed the Eighth International Congress of Applied Chemistry and announced, "Those who pay careful attention to their tastebuds will discover in the complex flavour of asparagus, tomatoes, cheese and meat, a common and yet absolutely singular taste which cannot be called sweet, or sour, or salty, or bitter . . ." Since that "absolutely singular taste" couldn't be assigned to any of the existing tastes, Dr. Ikeda christened his discovery "umami," which translates to "delicious" or "good taste." However, it wouldn't be until additional studies corroborated Dr. Ikeda's findings in the 1980s (nearly fifty years after Dr. Ikeda's death) that umami was internationally recognized as "the fifth taste." In 2008, the United States made such a big

---

6. Dr. Ikeda then patented the manufacture of monosodium glutamate, or MSG, that ubiquitous ingredient of Asian cuisine.

fat deal out of umami and what it suddenly meant to American cuisine (nearly a century after its discovery) that the Umami Information Center opened a branch office in New York with the goal of "raising public awareness of umami, disseminating the latest information to chefs, gastronomists, culinary schools and members of the media, and responding to queries."

All the tastes detected by the tongue have taste receptor genes associated with them that determine how the various tastes are perceived. The specific bitter taste receptor gene that Dr. Reed and her team would be extracting and analyzing after receiving my cheek swabs is known as TAS2r38. Just like with all our genes, we have two copies of TAS2r38, one copy from our mom and one copy from our dad. If the copy you get from your mom is the nontaster gene and the one you get from your dad is also the nontaster gene, you will not be able to taste PROP/PTC. If you get a taster and a taster, that makes you a supertaster for this particular taste receptor gene. Not only will you be able to taste PROP/PTC, but you will find it to be extremely bitter. If you get a taster and a nontaster, you will be caught in the middle as an average taster, meaning you will be able to detect bitterness, but it won't be that intense.

In order to keep me from spending hours with my nose pressed against the window waiting for my saliva harvesting delivery, I busy myself by exchanging informative emails with the exuberant and voluble Dr. Antti Knaapila, a postdoctoral fellow in Dr. Reed's group. Dr. Knaapila studies the genetics of adult food neophobia (the fear of trying new foods) at Monell, and to help me with some of my questions, he sends a few more scientific papers for me to peruse in my spare time.

When you're in search of very specific information, pawing through scientific papers is like disemboweling one of those Russian nesting dolls. The first article makes a claim and gives just enough information to be both intriguing and useless, unless you look up the source article behind that claim. The source article leads to another claim, and therefore another source article that needs to be looked up, and another and another until you finally reach the tiniest of all the dolls, which hopefully is where all the answers will be found since the tiniest of all dolls can't be opened. In this case, just one article from Dr. Knaapila leads to popping open twelve different multipage PDFs, and goes all the way back to man's discovery of fire. Literally.

Up until about eight hundred thousand years ago, Crog and Crug didn't have fire, and without fire, Crog and Crug couldn't cook. This meant that when it came to plants, Crog and Crug had a fairly limited diet. Various plants—some strains of acorns, potatoes, and parsnips, to name a few—may have tasted bitter and even been poisonous (or had very unfortunate gastrointestinal side effects) when scarfed down in their raw state. Eventually, the descendants of Crog and Crug learned how to cook or purify those plants to make them edible, while also noting that bitter taste was a warning sign. The most toxic elements that exist *in nature* taste bitter to humans. (I place particular emphasis on "in nature," because as most pet owners know, antifreeze tastes sweet to animals, and it's a very deadly sweet, but antifreeze is not a toxin that exists in nature—it is put together in a lab.)

Babies are biologically geared to be even more sensitive to bitter taste than adults. It might be because adult bodies with their mature organs and metabolic systems are better at detoxifying than brand-new, fragile baby bodies, and it also might be because babies explore and learn by putting everything in their mouths. Being naturally extra-sensitive to bitter taste is biology being a good baby-sitter. Bitter goes in, baby spits out.

The point is, having taste receptors that hone in on bitter tastes serves to protect humans from surrounding dangers. However, for those who have the misfortune to taste bitter too strongly, it also might prevent them from chowing down on bitter-tasting foods—such as kale and Brussels sprouts—that are actually good for them. At one point, Dr. Reed tells me, "[Bitterness] isn't necessarily 'no-go,' but 'slow as you go,'" adding, "Everything is a poison—it just depends on the dose."

When the cheek swabs finally arrive, I carefully undo the yellow Jiffy envelope,[7] slide out the plastic tubes that contain the swabs, and unfold a page of satisfyingly precise instructions from Amin Khoshnevisan, a senior research technician in Dr. Reed's lab. The instructions even tell me exactly how long each cheek needs to be swabbed! I love scientists.

Before I can get on with my swabbing, Mark, who overthinks things even more than I do, rushes over to stop me, explaining that it is the beginning of a hot holiday weekend. Meaning that if I were to swab and mail right now, my precious and possibly supertaster cells would sit in limbo until Tuesday. Would all of that heat and time degrade or denature the buc-

---

7. Seems like a very casual way of sending DNA collection materials, doesn't it? I was sort of expecting a metal box that hissed fogs of dry ice when I opened it. Because I watch too much TV.

cal cells? ("Buccal" sounds like a $12 plate of Mario Batali's house-cured meat, but it means "cheek.") Over email, Amin reassures me that my cheek cells are perfectly safe; according to Dr. Reed:

> DNA is remarkably stable—recall that Neanderthal DNA could be purified and PCR amplified. The rationale for keeping DNA samples on ice—or frozen—is not so much to protect the DNA from degrading, but rather to reduce the growth of bacteria.

Cool.

Armed with such knowledge, I was then able to have this conversation with my husband a few hours later:

Me: Should I scrape my cheeks tonight?

Him: Did you brush your teeth recently?

Me: Mark, tartar control toothpaste is not going to alter my DNA.

When I finally sit down to collect my DNA, Mark makes me read the instructions aloud before he allows me to uncap the plastic tubes holding the long swabs. After hearing that I need to swab each cheek for 30 seconds, Mark goes to the kitchen and comes back with the timer, which he places in front of me. Of course.

Once my buccal cells are safely in the mail, all I can do is wait. Some more. At one point I get a very tantalizing email from Dr. Reed telling me that her assistants have "extracted [my] DNA." It's totally going to come out that I'm the murderer of the week on *CSI*. Finally, finally, finally, I get the definitive email from Dr. Reed telling me that I am not, by any means, a supertaster. Nor am I an undertaster. What I am is average. I'm an average taster. It's what the Sweet'N Low Test told me, it's what the Blue Tongue Test told me, it's what the taste test strips told me, and it's even what the speed dating questionnaire on BBC.com told me. I'm average, and I'm even gladder that I didn't shell out $500 for 23andMe .com to tell me that.

In scientific terms, I'm heterozygous ("het" is the even cooler way to refer to it around the lab) for the TAS2r38 gene. If I had inherited two taster genes or two nontasters, I would have been homozygous. However, I got one taster gene from one parent and one nontaster gene from the other. Given how they reacted to the taste test strips, I'm assuming Mom gave me the taster and Dad gave me the nontaster.

Genetic Test Results: AVERAGE TASTER, NOT A SUPERTASTER IN ANY WAY, SHAPE, OR FORM. NOPE. NO. NU-UH.

Although I have checked *The Complete Idiot's Guide to Decoding Your Genetics* out of the library in order to cross "understand genetics" off the yellow stickie that serves as my research to-do list, I still don't quite comprehend what exactly goes on during the genotyping process. I confess I have this image in my head of scientists hunched over microscopes, looking at a slide smeared with my carefully scraped buccal cells, unraveling my lengths of DNA until they find the chromosome where the TAS2r38 gene lives.

After a morning when I deluge the very patient Dr. Reed with emails asking if the attached videos are accurate portrayals of the way they genotype at Monell, Dr. Reed breaks down and hands me the second-biggest high of this project: She invites me to come to Monell and work for a few days in the lab to learn the process for myself. Work! Me! IN A LAB!

Wait, me? Work? In a lab? I barely got through chemistry and AP biology. I managed to skip physics entirely—something that still confounds my almost-physicist, actual-mathematician husband—and I have chemistry class nightmares to this day.

After accepting her invitation, I felt the need to make it very clear to Dr. Reed that I am just a food writer and that I have no—zero, zip, zilch—science background. (Not that she can't already tell that from all my, "Duh, what's a gene?" questions, but I make sure to hammer the point home.) Did she still want me under those circumstances? "No worries," Dr. Reed wrote back cheerfully. "There is a saying in the lab that 'molecular biology is Chinese cooking,' which will make more sense to you once you visit and learn to pipette." And with that, I start making arrangements to spend five days at the Monell Chemical Senses Center in Philadelphia, where I'll be trading 70° and sunny for 30° and slushy, where I'll be learning how to genotype, and where, I hope, there will still be a lab standing after I leave.

CHAPTER 2

DNA Camp

Weeks before my trip, Mark starts bugging me to bring either his or Henry's DNA to Philly for analysis. I tell him I don't want to press the Monell folks since they have already been so generous with me. "I just think you should at least *ask*," he persists as he files dinner plates in the dishwasher. "They could send more swabs!" I squirm. He knows full well I don't like to impose on people. "I'm sure they have plenty of DNA there," I say. He looks me in the eye, and asks, "Because they just keep it around?" "Because it's their *job* to keep it around?" I point out, rather pleased with my logic. "I just think you should ask," he says, going back to his original argument. I muse this over and suggest, "Well, I guess I could ask in a way that doesn't sound like I'm just using them as our family's personal genotyper. I could email something like, 'If you need me to bring DNA with me, I could always—'" "Yes," Mark chortles, imitating me, "'I was packing and I was wondering if I should leave room for DNA.' No, no—go ahead, ask the right question, and you *will* sound dumb."

Guess who's not getting his DNA analyzed.

*

The night I arrive in Philadelphia, I get a text from my friend Catherine in San Francisco. "Don't burn down the lab!" it advises. Sound advice. I was two-thirds successful in packing for East Coast winter weather. I have my shiny red polka-dotted waterproof boots, and Catherine's puffy jacket. But on my first day of DNA Camp, Philadelphia is hit with a freezing rainstorm, and I realize what I don't have is an umbrella. Clearly, my six soaking wet winters in Boston had completely slipped my mind. Monell is only two blocks from the hotel, but it is still enough time outside to ensure that I spend the rest of the day in vaguely damp corduroys.

Big and solid, the Monell building in West Philadelphia's University City looks exactly the way you'd expect a science center to look: nondescript and kind of boring. However, the center's dull exterior most definitely belies the fascinating work being done inside. Imagine, a place solely devoted to understanding how we smell and taste! It's like Willy Wonka's Chocolate Factory . . . for people who really like tasting and smelling. Founded in 1967 by Dr. Morley Kare, a junior professor in (of all things) the veterinary school at Cornell, the center grew from humble beginnings into, according to their website, "the world's only interdependent, nonprofit scientific institute dedicated to research on the senses of taste and smell." Unique for its time, the center promotes interdisciplinary collaboration among psychologists, biologists, chemists, neuroscientists, and geneticists in order to fully understand these senses and their effects on everything from chronic disease and obesity to fragrance perception, homeland security, and pollution. Originally housed in an old bindery building owned by the University of Pennsylvania, the center and its approximately 60 PhD-level scientists now occupies a 60,000-square-foot building as well as adjacent property.

After all those emails of questions and answers and planning and questions and questions, my first face-to-face meeting with the diminutive Dr. Reed—"Call me Dani," she insists, pushing back the cloud of thick dark hair hovering around her face—still offers up a boatload of surprises on the supertaster front. All this time I've been experimenting on myself to see if I am a supertaster, I've been thinking that TAS2r38 is the *sole* bitter taste receptor gene. The one, the only, the single gene that would determine my supertastiness. My stint at DNA Camp teaches me that TAS2r38 is one of twenty-five bitter taste receptor genes! *One!* Not only that, but TAS2r38 is responsible for how we perceive the bitterness in a certain subset of bitter compounds—the compounds that are chemically similar to PROP and PTC and are found in Brussels sprouts, cabbage, and kale—but not *all* bitter compounds. From all the news, pop culture, and food articles I have read about supertasters, it sounded like TAS2r38 was the be-all and end-all gene for all possible bitter tastes. Not so. TAS2r38 deals with some bitter tastes, but not all. Science has also located another bitter taste receptor gene—TAS2r19—which is responsible for how we perceive quinine, the bitter stuff that makes tonic water taste so refreshing. Learning about the quinine gene didn't just blow my mind; it also forced me to abandon my new marital trump card.

After I had determined via the taste test strips that Mark was an undertaster, I would trot out his results as the parting shot of various disagreements. One day, he was foolhardy enough to refute my claim that putting the box of peppermint Joe Joe's cookies next to the box of Annie's cheddar bunny crackers made the cheddar bunnies taste like peppermint. "They do *not* taste like peppermint!" Mark mumbled through a mouthful of bunnies.

"Do too!"

"Do *not*!"

"Oh, what do you know anyway?" I countered. "You're an *undertaster*!" He had no comeback.

However, after learning about TAS2r19 and quinine, I can no longer tell Mark he's an undertaster. As Dani explains it, there are two genetic components to the TAS2r38 gene perceiving PROP. There's the on-off switch, and there's the volume. A taster's TAS2r38 switch, like rosé-swilling Rachel's, is turned on, and the volume is at 11. (The scientific community doesn't like the term "supertaster" and just uses "taster," "nontaster," and "het.") My TAS2r38 switch is turned on, but my volume is maybe about halfway up. Mark's switch on his TAS2r38 gene might be turned off, which would make him a nontaster/undertaster for PROP, but because his TAS2r19 switch is turned on, making him a taster for TAS2r19, he can taste the bitterness in quinine. In fact, he loves the bitterness of quinine.

In order to demonstrate how she, like Mark, can't detect PROP, Dani nudges a tiny plastic measuring cup of clear liquid across her desk to me. She lifts a second cup up to her lips and toasts, "To your health!" before tossing her shot off without a grimace. I raise my dose to my lips and take a more tentative slurp. Gah! I had been expecting bitter, but that is awful! It's *revolting*! I pull gulps from a water bottle and gasp that my reaction to the taste test strips had not been nearly as melodramatic. Dani gently explains that the taste test strips aren't that reliable. Dani and her crew have used the strips on people whose outcome they actually knew—because they had already extracted and analyzed the DNA—and had the strip results not always match the DNA results. Dani points out that the chemicals on the paper strips probably degrade over time.

But back to the earth-shattering information that we have twenty-five bitter taste receptor genes. All of these receptor genes have been found, and Dani explains that geneticists can look at the individual structures of these bitter taste receptor genes and see where people differ. However, what they don't know yet are the keys that unlock all of them. For instance, the key to unlocking TAS2r38 and getting a reaction from the human subject is PROP, and the key to unlocking TAS2r19 is quinine. What scientists don't know at this time are the keys to the other twenty-three, or whether or not some have keys that are related to one another. But they're working on it.

What is becoming clear to me at DNA Camp is that TAS2r38 isn't the only bitter taste receptor gene that matters. During one of my many Q&A sessions with Dani, I venture that one could still be considered a supertaster for other taste receptor genes. Okay, so my switch for TAS2r38 is turned on, but my volume isn't all the way up, but what about my volume on TAS2r19? I can taste quinine, so I know that my TAS2r19 is turned on, and the way I figure it, if that volume is at 11, I'm a supertaster, right? Dani dashes those hopes by explaining that their research has shown that when a person's switch for TAS2r38 is turned on and the volume is all the way up, that volume control often reflects how they react to other tastes, too. Possibly even how they react to textures and temperatures. Although, she counters, it's also true that they've found people who can't taste PROP (like Mark, their switch for TAS2r38 is turned off), but they report extreme reactions to other taste qualities. There's always a loophole!

Oh, and here's another thing: There aren't just five tastes—sweet, sour, salty, bitter, umami/savory—there are actually six. That's right: Along with our twenty-five bitter taste receptor genes, there are six tastes. The sixth taste is calcium/mineral, and not a ton is known about it thus far. When I explain this taste revelation to Mark over the phone one night, he asks, "So, is that what you taste when you lick a rock?" Not being in the habit of licking rocks, I don't know how to answer that, so I decide to ask Dr. Antti Knaapila what he thinks calcium/mineral tastes like. "For me, it's a little bit like fat-free milk . . . it makes that association," he tells me in his soft, low voice. That sort of makes sense, the idea that you might be able to taste calcium in skim milk, because often what people detect in higher-fat milks is the flavor of fat. As a substance, fat also has the ability to coat your tongue and soften or mask other flavors, so when you significantly reduce the fat as you do in skim milk, you might taste calcium instead. But since I'm all about experiencing things for myself at DNA Camp, I wheedle Dani into giving me a sample of the calcium solution from her minibar of tastes. My exact reaction: "Oh, that's weird." Dani laughs at me, "Yes, yes, indeed!" "I would not know how to describe it," I say slowly. "Except that it is . . ." "Something," Dani supplies for me. I nod. "Sour," I go on, "but a bit of bitter. But there's also a"—I clack my tongue around my mouth—"a mouthfeel there, like a roundness." "That's a typical descriptor," Dani says. "It's not bad," I say, still trying to puzzle it out. "It's clearly not sweet. Wow. That's weird." So that's what I can personally tell you about this new sixth taste: It's weird.

On the fourth day of DNA Camp, I get into the lab. (Okay, that's not exactly true, I have been in the lab every day, because that's where my desk is, but now I'm finally getting the chance to do more in the lab than just review my notes.) Every morning at DNA Camp, I crack open my laptop on my temporary desk, which is connected to, but slightly lower than, the tall lab counters. The lab counters and my desk are topped with a black slate-like material. It's like sitting at a chalkboard, on which my nervously damp fingers leave smudges that I habitually polish away at the end of the day. Directly upon entering the lab, there are a bunch of white lab coats hanging on hooks and one baby blue coverall suit with a hood. It looks vaguely like something you'd wear in a hazmat situation, except the coverall material feels as thin and papery as a doctor's examining room gown. Fingering the flimsy coverall, I wonder when I get to don all the mad scientist gear and list my dream wardrobe out in my head. Of course, there'd be the white lab coat, and probably rubber gloves, and a surgical mask to keep me from breathing all over the DNA. But there would also be a shower cap thing for my hair and two more shower cap things for my shoes. Maybe there would even be special goggles lest I get a contaminant in my eye and have to use the green eyewash station in the corner.

At the moment, the lab is quiet, and aside from a scientist a few rows away, I am the only one here. I look around at all the contraptions. Down the counter from my desk, a small cabinet with a glass door makes a grinding noise as it tips plastic tubes back and forth. I creep closer to find out what this thing was. I giggle. It's called a Shake 'n' Bake Hybridization Oven.

Anna Lysenko, one of Dani's lab techs, who, specifically for my benefit, presented an overview of DNA extraction and genotyping at a lab meeting the previous day, walks into the lab and starts assembling things at her station. I snap my laptop closed and wait expectantly. Today, at long last, was genotyping day!

Anna holds out a box of latex gloves to me. They are lavender, not the usual blue. I comment on this as I pull out a pair. Anna, her bright blue eyes lit with delight, tells me how excited she was to use lavender gloves when she started at Monell a few months ago. "Every other lab I worked in had the blue ones," she says, shaking her head.

As I work my hands into lavender rubber gloves, which gets harder as my hands conveniently start sweating from the effort, I ask Anna hopefully if she ever wears a lab coat. Perched on a tall stool at her station, getting all the components ready to extract DNA, Anna explains she wears a lab coat only when she works with her mice colonies, "Because they might pee on me and they smell really bad." Anna takes in my disappointment that the gloves—pretty, pretty purple though they might be—are going to be the entirety of my lab ensemble and grinningly offers to take a photo of me in a lab coat for my scientist mom's benefit. Thinking how far and wide that photo would travel once my mom got ahold of it, I demur.

Sarah Lipchock, a postdoctoral fellow at Monell, soon joins us at Anna's station. Huddling a mug of hot tea in her hands, she leans back against the counter and watches our progress while also answering all my fussy questions. What becomes incredibly clear to me over the few days I spend with her is that Sarah is a very good teacher. She, like Dani, is the kind of teacher who cuts right through the confusing science jargon and makes everything as clear as nuclease-free water. Sarah's current work at Monell involves a hunt for bitter blockers—substances that can prevent people from tasting bitterness. Salt, she explains, is one example of a bitter blocker. Naturally, my mind leaps immediately to how bitter blockers would make it easier for supertasters to eat the bitter-tasting healthful greens that they would normally find repugnant, but Sarah is specifically interested in finding bitter blockers to use in children's medicines. The AIDS cocktail in particular is horribly bitter, and trying to get kids to take this crucial medication is very difficult. Sarah explains that kids with the heterozygous TAS2r38 genotype (which is what I am, an average taster) are much more sensitive to bitter than their mothers who have the same genotype. "And adolescents are intermediate," she continues. "Something happens over the course of your lifetime that makes you much less sensitive to bitter, and we don't know what that is."

Earlier I asked Dani if these lifetime changes are due to our taste buds dying as we age, a popular explanation for why people suddenly find themselves liking foods that they hated as kids. Dani explained to me that our taste buds are composed of many cells, so the question really should be: Do taste *cells* die? Dani elaborated, "Taste cells have a ferocious cell cycle and probably turn over every ten to fourteen days. Your taste cells are not like your neurons, where once you have them, you're stuck with what you have." Eventually, Dani said, the taste cells probably do die and don't regenerate, just as with aging auditory and vision cells.

However, there haven't been a lot of studies performed where cells are actually extracted and counted. Instead, the science community goes by the number of papillae, which is a crude proxy for cell number. Dani continued that when people say their "taste" has changed, it's like saying their taste in music or their taste in art changed, "Because certainly people's *preferences* change as they get older, for reasons that are cultural and [due to] maturation. It's not as much a function of your sensory apparatus as much as people probably think. Like, does your taste in music change because your hearing decreases or does your taste in music change because you finally understand Wagner for the first time?"

Back in the lab, I finally get as much of my hands into the pretty purple gloves as is going to fit, and Anna hands over two long cotton swabs and tells me to swab my cheeks. Without Mark standing over me with the blue IKEA kitchen timer, I forget that I'm supposed to scrape and swab for thirty seconds. I end up swabbing for probably half that amount of time. One of the swabs comes out tipped with brown. I think it's from my breakfast Clif Bar. Good thing DNA extraction includes a process that removes impurities. Following Anna's instructions, I carefully dunk my swabs in the clear liquid Quikextract that Anna has added to little plastic tubes called Eppendorf tubes. I snap the flip tops of my Eppendorf tubes closed and move on to using my first lab contraption, the Vortex. When the base of the tube is pressed onto the rubber pad of the Vortex, the machine vibrates crazily, shaking up whatever is inside the tube. After we Vortex our Eppendorf tubes, which leaves my hand feeling silly and tingly from the vibrations, we put the Eppendorf tubes in a heating block. The Quikextract, Vortex, and heating block all work to burst open the cheek cells, releasing and isolating the coveted DNA. A component of the Quikextract also stabilizes the DNA and prevents it from degrading.

As my cheek cells simmer away in the heating block, I suggest to Anna and Sarah that there is a sure killing to be made from turning lab equipment into kitchen equipment. I tentatively tell them of my dream of having a burette in my kitchen that would titrate oil drop by drop and thus result in perfect homemade mayonnaise. I even wonder aloud if there's a place in my kitchen for the Vortex. I could use it to recombine a vinaigrette that had separated in the fridge. I have a feeling they're going to think I'm completely insane. Sarah jumps right in and tells me she wants a heat-and-stir plate for her kitchen. Mystified, I ask what that is. Sarah explains, "It's just a plate, and you put a magnetic bar in your solution, and there's a magnet in the plate that makes it stir, so it stirs your solution for you and it heats it up—wouldn't that be awesome in the kitchen?" Totally.

Anna moves to the next step in DNA extraction, which is to suspend the DNA in alcohol. Alcohol washes the DNA and purifies it. (I'm going to start using that as a reason to have another drink. "More Pinot, please—I'm purifying my DNA!") I ask Anna if she has any lab-to-kitchen dreams. Anna, who was born in the Ukraine but speaks English without any trace of an accent, tells us that, first and foremost, she wants a larger apartment with an actual kitchen, adding, "I'm really, really trying to justify getting a Kitchen-Aid mixer. In Ukraine, we never had any fancy cooking equipment. I don't know how to use a carrot peeler. I peel my carrots with a knife and I peel my potatoes with a knife because I've never in my life been exposed to a peeler." Sarah laughs incredulously that she would lose half the potato if she tried to peel with a knife. Anna gestures helplessly as though using a peeler and shrugs. "I have friends who come over for dinner, and they want to help, and I'm like, 'Yeah, can you peel these potatoes and carrots?' and they're like, 'Where's your peeler?' and I'm like, 'Never mind, I'll do it myself.'" She throws up her hands helplessly.

At this point Anna, who can't get a carrot peeler to work for her, explains that we're going to take the DNA out of the heat block and quantify it using a spectrophotometer and a nanodrop. I'm sorry, I know I see *Star Trek* everywhere, but come on—this IS *Star Trek*! "Mr. Spock, could you please use the spectrophotometer to quantify life on the planet below before we nanodrop in on them?"

What we're actually going to do with the spectrophotometer and nanodrop, now that we've isolated it and gotten rid of all the extraneous cellular crap we don't want, is see how much DNA we have by shooting light through a drop of DNA. The DNA absorbs light, and the nanodrop puts the absorbed light in the UV visible range. We will then look over at a laptop and check a graph that shows where the DNA peaked, which allows us to determine how much DNA we have. Anna hands me a plastic-tipped pipette and invites me to squirt my sample onto the nanodrop platform. I'm supposed to get the single drop of liquid right on this tiny black dot on a quarter-sized metal platform, and my hand is shaking. It takes me several tries to get it right, but Anna is nothing but calm encouragement.

Once we know how much DNA we have in our sample, we add a few more things that will bring in the necessary components for the replication and genotyping. One is a fluorescent pink substance called an SNP assay, which helps to amplify the particular area (the base pairs, if you remember your high school biology) of the gene we want to see. The other is an indigo fluid called the Taqman MasterMix assay. The Taq contains everything needed to make replication happen and also helps to essentially dye the specific part of the gene (again, the base pairs) that will tell us whether the subject is a supertaster, an average taster, or a nontaster. "I have the prettiest assay, I think, in all of Monell," Anna muses as she squirts indigo fluid from her pipette. Anna's appreciation of lavender lab gloves and indigo assays is outstripped by her love for the confocal microscope in the basement. Rolling her eyes in ecstasy, she waxes rhapsodic over this fluorescent microscope that "allows you to pick out specific parts of tissue you want to look at."

"It's powered by fairy dust," she informs me, pulling out a well plate, which is a square piece of hard plastic punched with rows of tiny wells. We use our pipettes to fill those holes with our template (the combination of the Taq, SNP assay, nuclease-free water, and quantified DNA) and slide it into the thermal cycling machine. Everyone's seen a well plate, because every time the news does a story on something in the science community, they roll stock footage of a lab tech filling well plates with a pipette. Well, today, I am that lab tech. After the thermal cycling machine does its thing, it blurts out its results on a laptop screen. Once we consult the plate map we made ahead of time (and by "we," I mean "Anna"), documenting which tiny well holds whose DNA, we can see who is a supertaster, nontaster, or average taster. Or in scientific terms, who is a taster, nontaster, or het.

On my second day of genotyping, Anna lets me use the multichambered pipette to fill a 96-well plate. This pipette looks like a metal chisel tool pastry chefs use to shave bits of chocolate off a huge block. Instead of the pipette ending in a single tip where the liquid squirts out in a single emission, the bottom of the pipette branches left and right like a hair pick, so multiple emissions can be squirted simultaneously. It's totally fancy. As I awkwardly try to siphon up stuff with the multichambered pipette, I ask Anna if her hand ever gets tired of the constant pipetting her job requires. The force needed to manipulate the button at the top of the pipette is not insignificant. Anna tells me her hand got pretty sore at one point, and her doctor advised her to stop using the pipette. Anna raises her eyebrows to show me what she thinks of that advice. "Can you only do it with your one hand?" I ask, looking at how she was deploying the pipette with her right hand. "No, I can use my left hand—I was born a lefty, but I was born in the Soviet Union, so my parents had to force righty on me, because it wasn't allowed. Because, like, lefties were the devil or something." Anna goes on that if you entered first grade as a lefty, the teachers beat your hand with their rulers until you became a righty.

Though immensely informative and well worth the trip to a wintry and wet East Coast, my days at Monell and a second analysis of my freshly scraped cheek cells don't change the results of my genotype. I am not a supertaster; I am het, an average taster. I will have to find another body part to blame for my pickiness.

My later attempts to describe the genotyping process to Mark come out like this: *"You scrape your cheek. Then, you add stuff to the scrapings, shoot light through it, add more stuff, stick it in an oven, and BAM! You are genotyped!"* Mark sighs, puts on his professor voice, and once again tries to help me. Marrying a scientist has totally paid off for my career. When I was a television recapper, Mark gave me the ammunition to bitch and moan every time the show *Star Trek: Enterprise* got the science horribly wrong. Now he takes digital photographs of my blue tongue to facilitate a counting procedure and dumbs down DNA extraction and analysis to a level even I can grasp. Although, at one point, he tries to explain "precipitate" to me, and since I keep trying to relate everything to cooking, he finally asks me, "It's like, how do you get the sugar out of sugar water?" "Don't put it in there in the first place!" I retort. Mark walks out of the room. "Undertaster!" I yell weakly after him.

Except that he's not. And I'm definitely not a supertaster. Slowly dawning on me is the realization that while it is appealing to think that, had I been a supertaster, I could have grandly waved away plates of strong fish and sauced offal and excused myself by saying, "I'm a supertaster" the way one might say they are the Queen of England or Batman, it still would not have explained a whole lot about my brand of picky eating. After all, while I can taste it, bitterness is not the thing that makes vegetables, bananas, raisins, hot cereal, and organ meats so repulsive to me. In fact, what bugged me most about certain foods as a kid was not that they were bitter, sweet, sour, salty, umami, or calcium-y—it was their texture. Their smell. Their flavor . . . which isn't the same thing as taste and is much, much harder to understand.

CHAPTER 3

Picky Eaters Have Common Sense

My mom has the uncanny ability to smell cat pee. Anywhere. So finely honed is her ability that she can smell cat pee *even where none exists*. Our house in Minnesota has played host to a long, swish-tailed parade of adored cats, and most of them were male. Now, while it is true that every single one of these male cats was "fixed," some still felt the need to mark their territory in the house. They did this usually in corners, and usually on carpets. The biggest problem with territory marking is that once one cat does it, every other cat that comes along feels the need to overmark that other cat's smell with his own. It becomes a veritable piling on of pee. Because of this and because of the amount of time she spent on her hands and knees applying various Stench-Be-Gone miracle cures to the formerly white shag carpet in the dining and living rooms, Mom has been known to walk into a room, sniff the air violently, and ask, "Is that cat pee? Did Nutsy *do something* in here again?" Since we never could smell what got her nostrils in such a violent quiver, my sister and I would mutter under our breath that the only place she smelled cat pee was up her own nose.

For many years now, I have been obnoxiously confident that I have a highly developed sense of smell, and I assumed I inherited this sensitivity from my cat-pee-sniffing mother. I have always been able to smell things my husband cannot, the faintest waft of an odor I hate has the power to make me nauseous, and walking into a house where spinach or squash is being prepared can set off a chain reaction of the most unattractive gagging.

I think about this as I meticulously stipple concealer around this, my most sensitive of organs, and get ready for another day at Monell Chemical Senses Center. You see, today is Smell Day at DNA Camp. Not only am I going to take something called a Sensory Ability Test (SAT), but I am also meeting with faculty members from Monell's olfactory department.

My first meeting is with Dr. Charles (Chuck) Wysocki, a lanky neuroscientist with kind eyes and a relaxed manner, who schools me in some odiferous basics before moving on to pickier subjects. I barely finish fumbling with my Dictaphone on the conference room table when Chuck leans back in his chair and makes a crucial point: Taste and flavor are two different things.

In the context of the sensory workings of the human body, taste applies exclusively to the aforementioned five: bitter, salty, sweet, umami, and sour. (Six, if we're starting to count calcium/mineral.) When winos slurp down a golden mouthful of Albariño and exhaustively soliloquize about undertones of peach and notes of honeysuckle, they're not talking about taste, they are talking about flavor. We perceive flavor when the senses of taste and smell join forces in the mouth, and the sense of smell actually plays the dominant role.

To get a more complete picture of this, take the jellybean test. Pinch your nose closed and without looking at the color of the candy, pop a jellybean in your mouth and chew it, but don't swallow. What do you detect? A crunchy, slightly sticky, and gelatinous texture, the temperature of the jellybean, and the taste of something sweet. Nothing else. Next, release your nose and continue chewing. Suddenly, you are inundated with a lot more sensory information. Maybe your mouth is tweaking with the now recognizable flavor of tart green apples or figuring out that the fatty-sweet taste is buttered popcorn, the weirdest jellybean flavor ever invented. When your nose is not engaged, you can still perceive the six tastes, so in the case of the jellybean, you can perceive sweet. But it's the sense of smell's sensory input that floods the mouth with what is recognized as *flavor*. So when people say they've lost their sense of taste to a cold, what they've actually lost is their sense of smell, and with that, they've lost their ability to detect flavor.

According to Chuck, by plugging your nose, you are preventing air that would normally flow from the back of the mouth up through the nose and out the nose. That particular airflow route is called "retronasal." "Orthonasal," Chuck explains, "is sniffing it." He sniffs loudly, waving one hand up to demonstrate. For instance, when people smell diesel behind a belching bus, they aren't claiming they taste the exhaust in their mouths. "That's [*sniff*] orthonasal—they know they are experiencing it that way. However, as soon as they put something in their mouth, and they swallow and now experience the full [retronasal] aroma, [their reaction is]: 'Boy, that *tasted* good!'" Chuck laughs, shaking his head. "Everybody makes that mistake, even professional chefs."

Our assumption that flavor perception occurs only in the mouth is not our fault exactly. When the aroma of something is being experienced in the mouth, the brain sneakily tricks us into identifying that entire experience as originating from the tongue. This happens, Chuck explains, because the taste system, the trigeminal system (the system of nerves responsible for sensation in the face), and the olfactory system all converge in the brain's frontal cortex. "The brain is basically saying, 'It's in the mouth, it's taste,' and that's where the confusion comes in." As for how exactly the brain interprets smells the way it does, well, Chuck tells me that science is still working on that mystery.

The human olfactory system is incredibly complex. Humans have about 450 olfactory genes that are currently in use, but other mammals have over 1,000. We probably used to have that many, too, but may have downsized thanks to evolution—as Chuck explains, "We're not on all fours with our nose close to the ground, paying attention to what's there." He pauses thoughtfully and continues, "Although if you force a person to do that, they can follow an odor trail."

"Have they . . . done that?" I ask tentatively. They have, and it was done at Berkeley. (Of course.) "Out in a public park area," Chuck adds, chuckling gently behind his bushy salt-and-pepper mustache. The experiment, which was conducted by Noam Sobel (the director of Berkeley's olfactory research program) and a graduate student, took barely three seconds to find on YouTube.[1]

Curious as to whether my particular mass of olfactory nerves, cells, and genes would astound Professor Noam Sobel, I ask Chuck if getting my problematic and enlarged adenoids and tonsils lopped off at the age of three improved my future perception of smell and flavor and therefore contributed to my descent into picky eaterdom. Like all scientists I try to buttonhole, Chuck is cautious in his response. "If the presence of the swollen adenoids or tonsils interfered with the retro-nasal delivery of odors, then yeah, it's possible." As for picky eating, "Each individual is likely different at the genetic level than his or her neighbor when it comes to the appreciation of odors, aromas. We don't know the full extent to which that genetic difference plays a role in the selection of cuisine, but it certainly may. We don't know what role it plays in forming a picky eater, but it may." Speaking of my mass of olfactory nerves, cells, and genes, I found out that they weren't so "astounding."

Earlier in the day, I sat down with Daniel Hwang, one of Dr. Reed's lab techs, so he could put me through an SAT, a smell and taste test that would help determine my level of smell and taste perception. For the taste portion of the test, I sipped from vials of clear liquid and tried to figure out

---

1. The video is called "Human Sniffer" and shows a woman clad head to foot in navy coveralls and white gloves. Over her ears she wears bulbous red noise-canceling headphones, and her eyes are covered with red fabric-enshrouded goggles to keep her blind. She crawls over the green grass, sniffing at the ground and following a scent trail of chocolate essence. I'll bet my mom could do that with cat pee.

whether I tasted bitter, sweet, salty, sour, or savory (umami). In one section of the test, I had to identify two different tastes in one liquid, and in another, I had to rank the strength of sweetness in five different vials. The ranking exercise was the most difficult. It was not hard to identify bitter, sweet, salty, sour, or umami, but trying to suss out which vial was sweeter or less sweet than another was practically impossible. Especially since I tossed each vial back like a shot and tried to rank them based on my memory of what the previous one tasted like. In retrospect, I can see that it might have been far more helpful if I had thought to take small sips from each vial, which would have allowed for repeated and informative side-by-side comparisons. "It's hard for me, too," Daniel said kindly.

When we got to the olfactory part of the test, I sniffed at another set of glass vials filled with clear liquid and tried to identify scents such as orange, cheese, vanilla, musk, milk, air, soap, urine, and alcohol. When I held the last vial under my nose, I smelled absolutely nothing, so I circled "air" as my choice. Tallying up my results, Daniel told me that the "air" vial contained galaxolide—a synthetic musk developed by chemists and fragrance companies—so if I had smelled anything, I probably would have described it either as soap or urine. Knowing this, I picked up the vial, determined to give it another go. It is a bizarre feeling to snort in air so hard that one of your nostrils actually pinches closed from the effort, yet not be able to smell something that is apparently giving off an odor. Wait! I smelled something! "Vinegar?" I offered. Daniel shook his head. Evidently my oh-so-sensitive nose was probably just picking up on trace amounts of the solvent they use to clean the vials.

In Dr. Reed's office, we discussed my SAT results and addressed my sadly malfunctioning nose, which wasn't malfunctioning at all. Just like with taste, when it comes to their interpretation of odors, each person is genetically different from their neighbor. Dani pulled down a glass vial from her minibar of tastes and smells and had me smell it. Again, I could detect absolutely nothing. "Oh, I smell something wonderful," Dani said, waving the vial under her nose and sniffing rapturously. Another vial she gave me smelled a bit like sandalwood or patchouli. "Something," I said, groping for an adequate description, "I'd find in an herb shop on Haight Street?" Delicately handling the bottle with the tips of her fingers, Dani wrinkled her nose and told me she smelled something horrible and couldn't bear to get it on her hands because then she'd smell it all day. The scent in question was androstenone, a steroid found in human sweat and urine and in boar saliva. Using androstenone, DuPont made something for pig farmers to use in their breeding practices. They called it "Boarmate." I kind of wish I hadn't been able to smell that.

Our opposite responses to the scented vials reminded me of an argument I innocently started on Twitter one day. I came home from the farmers' market with some paperwhite narcissus and (as you do) Tweeted about how much I adore their scent. My Twitter stream exploded. Carol responded, "Paperwhites and narcissus smell like farts," and Anita agreed that they were "gag-worthy." Jennifer Tweeted that, to her, narcissus have "such a sweet, round fragrance," but she worries about having company when hers are blooming because she knows how much some people hate them. While all this was going on, Mark walked into the kitchen, sniffed the air, and wondered who'd left the lid off the compost can. To him, narcissus smell like rotting garbage.

It's amazing how opposing reactions to floral scents can inspire such passionate—and in one case—even angry reactions. Albert Blakeslee, a geneticist, opened a booth at a 1935 New York City flower show to test people's reactions to the scent of freesias. "People practically got into fistfights over what they could and couldn't smell," Dr. Reed told me. Excuse me? Fistfights[2] over flowers? That was something I had to read. From an article written by Blakeslee called "Demonstration of Differences Between People in the Sense of Smell" and published in *Scientific American Monthly*:

> One woman, for example, before trying the flowers insisted that the whole affair was foolish. "Everybody knows that Freesias have a lovely odor and to ask if Freesias are fragrant is a silly question." It was suggested that she try the two varieties on the table herself and notice for a while how others voted. She started with the "A" flower and turned on us indignantly, "There is something the matter with these flowers, they don't smell at all! You have done something to them." She was assured that they had not been doctored in any way. As she put her nose down among the "B" flowers, her features relaxed and with a smile she exclaimed "A perfectly heavenly odor." While she waited watching the others, a man approached the "A" flowers

---

2. Of course, in the 1930s, it was "fisticuffs."

which she had been unable to smell and called them strong. Upon smelling the "B" flowers (Leucocoryne) which the woman had called heavenly, the man's features hardened and he turned to the attendant almost with anger and said, "Lady, these stink, they stink like h-." The objecting woman's face flushed and she left the group without further objections.[3]

I have a new understanding for why I always thought I was too unsophisticated to appreciate the smell of Chanel No. 5—I find it unbearably heavy and cloying—and I remember my older sister's incredulity when I told her what I thought of it. To her, Chanel No. 5 is clean and light. To me, it's what I imagine a migraine would smell like.

Except with the most familiar odors, it's actually quite difficult to blindly smell something and identify it without some sort of context. Sniffing your way down the hall, you might have reason to wonder, "What in god's name is that *smell*?" But when you get to the kitchen and see cabbage cooking away on the stovetop, you realize, "Yes! *That's* what I've

---

3. Blakeslee gets downright snarky in the article when describing a woman who passed up the chance to sniff freesia for his experiment: "A young lady of modern appearance, however, was heard to say that she didn't want to help science, science had never helped her. She had evidently been helped, but perhaps it was art rather than science that had had the most influence." In another less snarky but wittier example, Blakeslee reacts to a woman who didn't like the odor of the pink freesias because she hates the color pink. "And she left," Blakeslee writes, "without giving us an opportunity to record her olfactory reactions to the Freesias which had the misfortune to be born pink."

been smelling!" And suddenly, you wonder how you failed to recognize that odor right away. Your brain often needs some sort of hint in order to identify the source of an odor. Scientists call this hint "context and expectation."

Back in the Monell conference room overlooking the slushy streets below, Chuck tells me about a slick experiment he performs on professional food and wine writers and tasters to demonstrate context and expectation. The audience is given vials to sniff. Each vial contains a strip of filter paper dipped in butyric acid. The concentration of butyric acid is exactly the same in both vials. Chuck pauses and asks if I know what butyric acid is. I don't. "It's a short-chain fatty acid that smells—" Chuck stops himself, considering whether or not to tell me. "Well, I'll give you the example." Half of the vials are labeled "food," and the other half are labeled "body." Half of the audience smells the "food" vials and the other half smells the "body" vials. Neither half of the audience knows what the other half has written on their vials. When the food-sniffing portion of the audience is asked how many of them found the smell enjoyable, half of them raise their hands. When those that sniffed from the body vial are asked the same question, no one raises their hands. Chuck tells me that butyric acid can be interpreted as Parmesan cheese. "But," he continues, "if you put the label 'body' on it, it's nasty foot odor." He grins at me. "And that's just the cognitive influence. So you have bias, and you have expectation," Chuck says, ticking these off with his fingers. "Because you've been given a little bit of information—food or body—now your mind is set to interpret what you're smelling in a certain way."

While it doesn't stop me from loving the flavor of it, I personally think Parmesan cheese smells like vomit. And I can say that with the assurance of a professional, because I put in some hard hours at a pungent San Francisco cheese shop. Being a cheesemonger gave me access to hundreds of varieties, and it also inspired a songbook of cheese-based ditties I dubbed "Songs of Cheesus," featuring such classics as "God Rest Ye Merry Cheesemonger" and "O Christmas Cheese, O Christmas Cheese."[4] On the hottest days in the cheese shop, I was never repulsed by the smell of even our stinkiest cheese, but that's likely because I have always been a cheese fanatic. Not only is it my chocolate, but when I was growing up, grilled cheese sandwiches and Stouffer's macaroni and cheese are what kept me going through the picky years.[5] It's possible that Parmesan cheese doesn't repulse me because Janeane Garofolo pointed out its connection to vomit in the film *The Truth About Cats and Dogs* only after my brain had decided I loved it.

See, whether you smell vomit or cheese, once your brain has identified a smell and decided it doesn't like it, it's pretty difficult to convince it otherwise. A pattern has been set. When it comes to being grossed out by the smell of something inedible, you can simply pinch your nose and try to get out of range as quickly as possible. However, when it comes to

---

4. For the complete lyrics, go to www.grubreport.com/blueplatespecial/cheesecarols.html and sing along next Christmas.

5. No, it's not local, it's not artisanal, and it's only homemade because you actually do put the delicious frozen brick in your oven or microwave *at home*. However, Stouffer's set the standard for all macaroni and cheeses that were to come into my life, and I still stock it in my freezer.

food, you'll probably stop eating the food whose smell/ flavor—remember, your nose has everything to do with the food's flavor in your mouth—makes you gag or nauseous.

However, this negative pattern setting doesn't have to be permanent. In a *New York Times* article examining why so many people hate cilantro, Harold McGee wrote, "Every new experience causes the brain to update and enlarge its set of patterns, and this can lead to a shift in how we perceive a food." To a lot of people, cilantro tastes like soap. This interpretation occurs because when the brain encounters a new flavor, it goes through its archives, trying to access a previous experience with that flavor. Sometimes the brain doesn't find a food-related match and instead connects the flavor to, as the article says, "chemical cleaning agents and dirt, or crawly insects." When that happens, the brain sends out an alarm that whatever is in the mouth is dangerous, and a pattern of revulsion or dislike is set. But it is possible to reset this pattern. Dr. Jay Gottfried, a neuroscientist McGee interviewed, explained that while he didn't like the flavor of cilantro at first, he also didn't go out of his way to avoid eating it. Instead, he continued to eat dishes that contained cilantro and eventually came around to liking it. Dr. Gottfried hypothesized that enjoying these dishes in the company of friends and family helped change his associations with the herb and convinced his brain to reset the original pattern. It also helped that Dr. Gottfried liked the other ingredients in the cilantro-laced dishes. (Chapter 6 explains more about how our emotions affect the body's reception of food.)

Chuck tells me that he experienced a pattern reset with that summertime staple: lemonade. "When I was a kid," he says, "I totally refused lemonade. To me, lemonade smelled like skunk." And growing up in the countryside of central New York, Chuck smelled skunk a lot. "I couldn't understand why people were drinking lemonade." After spending a summer mowing lawns under the hot sun, teenage Chuck was thirsty enough to finally come around to drinking his mother's lemonade. "And I liked it! So, I had to admit if I like the smell of lemonade, I've gotta like the smell of skunks, and that's what I did—I came around." He reset that pattern of disliking lemonade, which, interestingly, also means that he likes the smell of skunks. It is not an offensive smell to him. "Does the smell of skunks make you thirsty?" I ask. Chuck laughs. "No."

It's right about here that I have a forehead-slap moment in my quest to discover the causes of picky eating and how I got past my own pickiness: I have experienced the pattern reset as well. Except I didn't realize it was a pattern reset. In telling people about how I nudged myself into the terrifying territory of fish, foreign grains, and vegetables, I've called it "exposure therapy." (Others might call it "stealing food off your husband's plate.") In the days when I was no longer picky but not fully converted either, I was in my experimental phase. I was open to new foods, but not so open that I would order a plate of them in a restaurant. It was less threatening for Mark to order them, because this would allow me to snag small bites from his plate without committing to an entire plate of my own. As I sampled things here and there—a wisp of sautéed chard here, a flake of firm white fish there—it dawned on me that I didn't mind these foods. As a matter of fact, I was not minding to the point of actually liking some of them, because they weren't as bad as I'd feared. This exposure therapy of mine led to a complete pattern reset for a large number of foods that, soon enough, I was bold enough to allow on my own plate.

A few weeks later, I'm speaking to Amy Watts—a recovering picky eater and librarian from Georgia—when I learn that I'm not the only picky eater who embarked on her own exposure therapy cure. Amy, like me, ate virtually no vegetables for many years. During those years, she had a particularly disastrous encounter with spinach that culminated in a dash to a restaurant bathroom to spit out her mouthful before she threw it up on her date. "I felt like such a failure as a human being right then," she confesses to me. After that, Amy decided that spinach was her personal demon and has now been making concerted efforts to exorcise it. Just a few days before our conversation, she made one such attempt, "And I ate one forkful. I ate two forkfuls, and in the third forkful I realized: This is going to be my last forkful. I can't eat any more of this tonight." But Amy is not giving up. Instead of forcing herself to eat great wads of the stuff, Amy is trying to like spinach by eating it in a variety of ways (in a butter-grilled sandwich, smothered by cheese), and by doing this, she is forcing a pattern reset.

I've overcome many of my food hates in a similar fashion: I doggedly chipped away at certain foods—tried them *in* things, tried them *on* things—until I liked them. In some cases, I fell head over heels for the food and ate it every night for weeks. (In other cases, I realized I would never really love, or even like, the food, but I could at least tolerate it.) For instance, I don't like big messes of greens. Whether we're talking beet greens, kale, spinach, or chard, I can't sit down and eat a bowl of them. It's their nearly tooth-resistant texture that bugs me more than anything else, because the unchewable food spends way too much time in my mouth, which risks triggering my gag reflex. However, when I hit upon the idea of chopping them up in manageable pieces, sautéing them with garlic, and adding them to pasta, brown rice, or farro—a method that helps break up the clumps of greens, providing a varied texture—I actually love them.

Amy and I aren't the only picky eaters who have issues with the way a food feels in the mouth. In Chapter 4, it is a texture question on the Duke Food F.A.D. Study survey that allows me to babble on at obscene length about "texture violations." The very existence of that texture question means the eggheads studying our unique eating habits are well aware that many picky eaters are bothered by the texture of food. In some cases, the abhorrent texture of the food—not the flavor—is the picky eater's main complaint. Amy is also repulsed by mushy foods like grits, oatmeal, and cream of wheat. "I don't like food that feels like someone else has digested it." However, it's not just slimy, regurgitated foods that gag picky eaters with a spoon. When it comes to how something feels against their tongue, teeth, and inside cheeks, there's a wide range of food textures that gives picky eaters the gut shudders. Some picky eaters can't stand food that is too crunchy or too chewy or too soft or too wet. And then there are those picky eaters who are extremely sensitive to temperature, like Julie Burba.

The way Julie bounced from kitchen to kitchen at our Boston-area culinary school told me all I thought I needed to know about her palpable relish for food and cooking. With snapping eyes brimming with delight above her food-smeared white chef's coat, Julie struck me as someone who never shrank from any kind of food. Divinity or offal, Julie seemed open to it all. I didn't remember that picky eaters—former or current—*look just like everyone else*. You could have knocked me down with a basil branch when Julie confessed to me on Facebook that she also had a picky past.

"I was a texture eater," Julie later tells me over the phone. "I didn't like the way food felt in my mouth. I wouldn't eat anything I thought was 'wet,' like a condiment. I couldn't stand the feel of sauces." Julie also didn't like things that would "pop" in her mouth, "Anything that was a weird experience for my mouth—that, I didn't like." She was particularly bothered by temperature extremes. If food was either too hot or too cold, it freaked her out, which was why bringing soup in a thermos was a lunchtime staple when she was growing up. By the time lunch rolled around, the soup had sat around long enough to become tepid, her ideal temperature. "Because I knew that I could drink it—it was more of a drinking kind of thing for me, rather than eating," Julie explains. It's not exactly a ringing endorsement for the thermos's raison d'être, but hey, it worked for Julie. These days, Julie is willing to try absolutely anything. While it used to be something that would prevent her from trying a new food, Julie tells me that today she doesn't even notice the textures or temperatures she once despised.

At this point scientists don't completely understand why texture aversion occurs, but they do think there might be a correlation between having an unusual sensitivity to the way a food feels and the way a food tastes. Dr. Marcia Pelchat, a faculty member at Monell Chemical Senses Center who studies how people respond to the sensations of food, explained that being exceptionally sensitive to food temperature is not uncommon among picky children. Via email, Dr. Pelchat explains that there is evidence that picky eaters are more sensitive to oral sensations (texture included) than nonpicky eaters, but not enough research has been done to determine the reasons why.

Fine, we don't know why, but we know texture violations happen and not just to self-aware picky eaters either. Plenty of people can relate to being turned off by textures. My mother-in-law, for instance, dislikes the mushy, gooshy feel of foods like bananas and grits. But she doesn't consider herself a picky eater. However, fixating on how much they loathe the texture that is currently rolling around in their mouth—if they've even managed to get that far—can stimulate something picky eaters are far too familiar with: the gag reflex.

"Wow, I'm impressed—you didn't gag," the University Health Services nurse commented as she pulled out the tongue depressor and rubbed the contaminated swab on a petri dish coated with pink jelly. I was a freshman in college, downed by some evil scourge that even the antiseptic effects of alcohol couldn't drive away. She asked if I was a vocalist, which struck me as an odd question until she explained that trained singers often have a very good command of their gag reflex. I hypothesized that maybe having my throat swabbed for so many strep cultures before I finally had my tonsils and adenoids removed must have accustomed me to the constant prodding and scraping. As it turns out, I wasn't just whistling Dixie on that one.

The roof of your mouth is made up of the hard palate in

the front and the fleshier soft palate in the back. Prodding, poking, touching, or even just grazing the soft palate, which is near the opening to the throat, is what goads the gag reflex (pharyngeal reflex) into action. The primary function of the gag reflex is one of pure protection, as it constricts to block any unwanted objects—foreign or domestic—from entering the throat. While the gag reflex can be stimulated by touch (somatic reaction), the stimulus can also originate in the brain (psychogenic reaction), where just the sight, smell, or thought of a piece of gaggable food is enough to get the gorge a-rising.

For some picky eaters, the gag reflex is the biggest hurdle to overcome because, once triggered, it can be incredibly difficult to suppress. Now while as a child, I gagged mightily as I washed down mouthfuls of string beans, succotash, and zucchini, I never actually threw anything back up. Given this decided lack of undigested physical evidence and judging by their eye rolls, I'm sure my parents were fairly certain that my tableside retchings were all sham gags, and wrote me off as the girl who cried puke.[6] If I could have just pulled off what my picky friend Keith did, who puked right at the table after being forced to eat peas when he was six, my parents might have been convinced.

Whether you are a hurler or not, the gag reflex presents quite the problem. After all, a reflex by definition is involuntary, so it's not exactly something most people have natural

---

6. In the interest of full disclosure, I did a fair amount of sham gagging on the nights I walked into the kitchen and found out that what we were having for dinner didn't meet with my picky approval.

control over. As an adult, I was too worried about offending people by not eating the food at their houses, so I had to find a way to shut my gag reflex up. What I found was that I could force my gag reflex into hibernation if I just tried really hard. (Surreptitious deep breathing and wine and chewing and swallowing as quickly as possible also helped the process.) "Just try really hard" is, however, completely pointless advice, so I decided to talk to people who deal with the gag reflex as part of their chosen career. (Go ahead and get all the knee-jerk porn star jokes out of your system, because that's not where I'm going with this.) As far as I'm concerned, the true masters of their gag reflex domain are professional sword-swallowers.

Sword-swallowing always struck me as some trick involving sleight of hand or perhaps a collapsible sword. It's not. "If you could fake it, Criss Angel would do it," the sword-swallowing Lady Aye tells me in an interview. It's all real. They really are sticking a sword down their throat, down their gullet, right to the opening of their stomachs. In some cases, the sword-swallower goes one step further and slides the metal blade *into* his stomach until it touches the organ's soft floor. Think about that for a minute. *Swords!* I still can't wrap my mind around that. I won't even eat raisins.

Obviously the very first thing sword-swallowers-to-be need to do—aside from making sure they have health insurance—is overcome their gag reflex. And apparently, you can find the ideal tool in your own closet. "The industry standard is a wire coat hanger," Todd Robbins informs me, "a traditional Joan Crawford memorial wire coat hanger." Todd is a New York performer who specializes in the weird and the offbeat. He earns his living by swallowing swords, eating lightbulbs, walking on glass, using his head to break cinder blocks, and teaching sword-swallowing at Coney Island. Todd explains that the best method is to stretch and bend the coat hanger until it forms the rough outline of a sword, approximating the sword's width and shape, "And then one morning before breakfast, because you sure as hell don't want to do it after breakfast, you stand—preferably in the bathroom—and throw your head back and try to find the correct alignment." Finding the correct alignment is difficult, which is why embryonic sword-swallowers start their training under the guidance of a seasoned professional. "There's really no flail factor in this. You do it right or you die," Todd adds.

(Just so we're all clear and no one out there goes and does anything ill advised at home, this chapter is not to be treated like Sword-Swallowing 101. If you want to go be a sword-swallower, that's just fine, but for goodness' sake, get professional instruction and training. Don't just start sticking long, sharp objects down your gullet willy-nilly.)

Todd explains that bypassing the gag reflex can take anywhere from two to six weeks if the sword-swallower keeps up their regimen. "You do what I refer to as seven-by-seven, which means you do it every day, seven times in a row for seven days." After the gag reflex is conquered, there's other internal training the sword-swallower needs to undergo—getting past the glottal opening, deciding if they want to go right to the bottom of their stomach or stay outside of it, choosing the right swords, etc.—but we're sticking with the gag reflex since that is what affects picky eaters.

According to Todd, while sword-swallowers might overcome the gag reflex where swords are concerned, they still do have a gag reflex, which will get triggered if it senses something that it doesn't want there and is therefore a threat. You know, something that is not a sword or a sword-shaped hanger. Something *abnormal*, such as cooked spinach or squash. This explains why I could handle getting my throat swabbed, but it still took me a while to stop gagging over certain foods. At some point, I just accepted the tongue depressor and the cotton-tipped stick and everything they needed to do to me. However, I still hadn't accepted that certain foods were okay. Similarly, Lady Aye admitted to me that she gags if she gets a little too energetic with her tooth brushing. Long metal swords that slide all the way down to the pit of her stomach—that, she can do. Toothbrushes, not so much.

You couldn't ask for a better segue than tooth brushing to move on to my next set of gag reflex experts: the "Are you flossing?" crowd. Since dentists deal with their patients' gag reflexes on a daily basis, I decide to make a fluoride-free appointment with mine.

Although I went for a cleaning barely a month before, I still feel strangely self-conscious about the state of my teeth when I meet with Dr. Nabai. I feel the same sort of self-consciousness when I run into my hair stylist on the street and my hair is scraped back into a ponytail with absolutely no regard for my bangs; it's like I'm not taking good care of their work. However, since Dr. Nabai doesn't open our conversation with, "Your gums look a little puffy," I push away thoughts of attempting to conduct the interview through a barely opened mouth.

Dr. Nabai tells me that many of her patients are bothered by their own toothbrushes, but she's read that it's possible to disengage the gag reflex by exposing it to constant stimulation. For instance, if brushing your way-back molars makes you retch and heave, just pushing your toothbrush slightly farther back each time could help accustom you to the sensation and quell the gagging. Dr. Nabai admits there are differing levels of sensitivity: "Some people are so sensitive, you touch the floor of their mouth and they start gagging, but for most people it's going to be their soft palate." While Dr. Nabai does have patients who are so sensitive they gag when anything goes into their mouth during a cleaning, it's making mouth molds that give patients—even the nongaggers—the most trouble. In some cases, Dr. Nabai applies a topical numbing gel to the soft palate, which helps quash a lot of gagging. The numbing gel Dr. Nabai uses is akin to but weaker than a numbing agent known as Hurricaine spray, which doctors use for some endoscopic procedures.

If you don't watch *Grey's Anatomy*, endoscopy is a procedure during which a tiny camera called an endoscope on a long lead is inserted into one of a patient's orifices. The Hurricaine spray is used to control the gag reflex when the patient is required to swallow the endoscope, like in a situation where their gastrointestinal tract needs to be checked out. The gag reflex is unsurprisingly not usually an issue when the endoscope is put in the opposite end of the patient for a colonoscopy. (Todd, the sword-swallower, told me he doesn't need those numbing sprays when he's had endoscopic procedures. He just deep-sixes that camera, no problem.)

For Dr. Nabai, numbing gel combined with keeping the appointments short and providing additional distractions, like the option to watch movies during the procedure, usually does the trick to keep the patient's gag reflex at bay. "Have you ever had a patient throw up on you?" I ask Dr. Nabai. "Oh, yes," she responds and adds that, in some cases, she might decide that a little whiff of nitrous oxide (laughing gas) might help the patient and their gag reflex relax even more.

Since picky eaters obviously can't and *shouldn't* use either numbing agents or laughing gas to get through a meal, I decide to investigate another antigagging tip that kept popping up on dental blogs and in dental papers. It's very simple, this one: Just breathe through your nose. More than anything else, breathing through the nose is a distraction for the patient. "It's nothing to do with anatomy, it's having the person focus on something else to take their mind off it," Dr. Dorothy Burk, the director of the gross anatomy course at the University of the Pacific School of Dentistry, tells me. She adds that some doctors have suggested that telling the patient to lift their legs can help, too. Clearly, lifting your legs has no anatomic connection to your gag reflex; it's merely another way to divert your attention away from what's going on in your mouth.

Since practitioners of yoga are also told to breathe through their nose to sharpen concentration and deepen relaxation as they attempt to contort their body into a braying serpent or release the tension in their earlobes, I suggest nasal breathing possibly achieves the effect of naturally chilling the gagging patient out. Dr. Burk agrees it might and tells me about the scientific papers that discuss the successful application of acupuncture for gag reflex issues.

I'm not an acupuncture skeptic. Quite the contrary, acupuncture has helped me combat recurring and mysterious vertigo as well as equally mysterious and also recurring side pain. However, the idea of those teeny, light needles working on a single point located right below the lower lip to quell such a strong reflex as a gag does raise my eyebrows. Those same eyebrows eventually lowered once I read a scientific paper documenting how acupuncture point CV-24 (the Conception Vessel Meridian[7]) was used to prevent the gag reflex while a dental impression was taken of the upper teeth. Even more compelling evidence is found in another paper that details how point CV-24 was used to control the gag reflex during a transesophageal echocardiography (meaning it was needled during a procedure where a camera was snaked down patients' throats and esophagi to take a look at the heart). That's a pretty impressive test of point CV-24's power, but it's not even the most mind-blowing example of what acupuncture can do. During one of our sessions, my acupuncturist tells me about a Bill Moyer special that showed a fully conscious patient having brain surgery where the only pain blocker used was acupuncture. "I don't think I'd have the guts to do that," I tell her. "Stephanie," my acupuncturist says as she flicks a needle into the skin of my hand, "I'm an acupuncturist, and *I* wouldn't have the guts to do that."

Unfortunately, much like the topical numbing agents and laughing gas, getting picky eaters to eat all their meals with a needle sticking out of their Sauce Receptacle isn't exactly practical. This brings us back to deep breathing and concen-

---

7. The Chinese name for this point is Cheng Jian, and the English is Sauce Receptacle, which is so awesome that I have to find a way to refer to my Sauce Receptacle as much as possible.

tration as the most helpful exercise in tableside gag reflex control. Admittedly, a lot of picky eaters might react to the touch or taste of a hated food in their mouth, but the psychogenic response is usually even more powerful in that it prevents the picky eater from even putting the food in their mouth in the first place. Case in point, just talking to my colorist about her lettuce and greens aversion gets her so agitated she starts fanning herself with her hand. "I'm getting all freaked out," she confesses as I duck streaks of plant-based hair dye.

In these psychogenic situations, aphorisms such as "mind over matter" or "it's all in your head" trip easily and lazily off the tongue. Bah! I prefer to quote Mr. Spock, who said, "Pain is of the mind. The mind can be controlled." I used to have a serious texture aversion to peaches, and the way I got past my gag reflex in a peach-heavy situation, where failure to ingest was not an option, was to take deep, measured breaths through my nose and to practice a little Vulcan mind control.

First of all, you should know that even in the best of situations, I'm not a calm houseguest. I'm nervous about being a nuisance. I obsess over showing proper yet not obsequious graciousness. I worry about waking anyone up in the dead of night when I have to get the glass of water I somehow didn't plan for when I went to bed. I fear overflowing the toilet for no reason other than the toilet chose that particular moment to get clogged up. When it came time to pay my first visit to my future in-laws, I was particularly worried about the toilet issue, because I'd be known as "that girl who clogged our downstairs toilet" until the very end of time. It wouldn't matter if I got married and gave them grandkids. I wouldn't be Mark's wife, their daughter-in-law, or the mother of their grandchildren. I'd always be "that girl who clogged our downstairs toilet." But back then, the thing that topped my Worried Houseguest list was food.

Mark was aware of *some* of my food hates and he dutifully warned his parents ahead of time that anything made with peppers was liable to migraine me to my bed and result in vomiting. (Which, in turn, would make me a nuisance, put my graciousness in a very dim light, and most definitely clog up the toilet.) Not knowing then just how deep my vein of pickiness ran, my peppers "allergy" was the only thing he thought he needed to warn them about. Peaches were not something he ever imagined would be a threat to my gag reflex.

As we all tucked into a wonderful dinner of leg of lamb that had been butterflied and grilled to pink perfection over rosemary smoke, Mark's dad raised his glass of Barolo and toasted our engagement, welcoming me into their family. Everything was pleasant, warm, and downright hunky-dory until Mark's mom brought out the dessert: peaches. They had been slipped out of their skins before poaching, so of course, they were peaches at their slitheriest. I swallowed hard, knowing there was no way out of this. I was not going to jeopardize my future in-laws' opinion of me by refusing this carefully made dessert. I had to eat whatever was in front of me. And what was in front of me was an amber moon of a summer peach, warmed by a spiced wine sauce. It sounds great when I describe it like that, right? But it was still a peach, and therefore evil. Cue the quiet nasal breathing. I was careful to take breaths that were deep enough to calm me down, but not so heaving that I would appear to be hyperventilating.

Smearing a politely intrigued smile across my face, I carved off a small section of fruit with the side of my spoon. As I watched garnet rivulets of the honey-thickened sauce coursing down the peach's soft flesh, I made mental peace with the fact that this piece of peach was about to enter my mouth, and I firmly instructed my gag reflex to back the hell off. And then I took two more surreptitious deep breaths. Finally, I popped the piece in my mouth and did a quick chew-chew-swallow. But soft, what delight in my mouth is this? It's true that angels in golden nightgowns didn't *exactly* trumpet from on high, and there weren't *reams* of doves soaring out of the fireplace to tie a big pink ribbon in my hair, but suffice it to say, not only did my gag reflex fail to make an appearance, I actually *liked* the piece of peach. I liked it so much, I took another bite and another. My peach pattern had been reset.

Me: 1; Gag Reflex: 0.

I was hooked, and not just on peaches, but on my mind games. Successfully subduing my gag reflex in this instance gave me the courage to try the same tactic on other foods to see what else I might be missing. In some cases, it worked and I discovered a new food obsession. Other cases: not so much. (I'm looking at *you*, bananas, you yellow-bellied sacks of slime-riddled stank!)

Taste, smell, and touch are all senses that have a great impact on a picky eater and their ever-present and ever-excitable gag reflex. But hang on, we're missing one of the senses here! (Technically, we're missing two, but I have yet to find a picky eater who took issue with the way a food sounded.) It would be negligent not to round out the discussion and talk about the importance of how a food *looks* to a picky eater, and Chapter 9 is where I posit my half-baked but totally compelling theory that picky eaters are both foodies in disguise and destined to ascend to a higher plane of existence—but first I have an identity crisis.

CHAPTER 4

The Picky Eater Has an Identity Crisis

"Well, you had a *moderate* problem with pickiness, but for the most part you've coped just fine."

After completing the questionnaire for the Food F.A.D. (Finicky Eating in Adults) Study, I am speaking to one of its architects, an eating disorder specialist. Who, as it turns out, is unconvinced about the debilitating trauma of my picky past. Well, maybe not "debilitating," exactly, but it really did suck there for a while. But "moderate"? Really?

Before clicking my way through the online survey and having my picky past called into question, I was pretty convinced the scientists behind the Food F.A.D. Study had never heard a story as fascinating as mine. In fact, as soon as I read about this collaborative study from Duke Medicine and the University of Pittsburgh Medical Center, I was enveloped in fantasies of becoming a breakthrough case study. The how and why were hazy, but I do know that it involved all the picky eater scientists standing around me in white coats and stethoscopes. "What a wonder she is," they would say, stroking their chins thoughtfully. "She ate practically *nothing* as a child and now look at her! Almost completely cured!" They would ask probing questions, draw blood and do brain scans, and eventually put on hazmat suits, tent my house, and attach long, covered tubes leading out to the street. (Apparently, my scientific daydreams are heavily influenced by *E.T.*)

Now it's true that I consider myself a recovering picky eater, but there was a time in my life when I dreaded food, which is exactly why I was so psyched to take the survey. For one thing, the Finicky Eating in Adults survey is the first of its kind, and how can anyone not want to be part of a groundbreaking study? Second of all, the results of the study will aid in the development of therapies that will help adult picky eaters, and since I know what it feels like to be an adult picky eater, I'm definitely keen to help others who are still dealing with it.

Little did I know that my participation in this groundbreaking study would call my own picky eating identity into question, something I'd assumed was a given.

It all starts when I read through one of the first pages of the survey, which presents a few "Does this describe you?" statements geared to make picky eaters shout, "Yes! That is me! I *am* one of these people! I AM SPROUTACUS!" For me, however, it has the opposite effect. Here, I'll show you what I mean:

I only eat white foods.

No one could accuse me of eating Joseph's Technicolor Dreamcoat in my picky prime, but I never was a monotone eater. In fact, there are a lot of beige foods I still openly hate.

I don't go out to dinner with friends because there is never anything I can eat.

Sure, there was a time when I sought refuge in the fried food-heavy kid's menus even when I hadn't been a "kid" for a decade, but going out to dinner is currently one of my favorite activities.

I find a lot of foods disgusting.

Um. What's "a lot"? Are succotash, raisins, bananas, oatmeal, cream of wheat, grits, polenta, the skin of tomatoes, caviar, offal, innards, feet, ears, flan, tofu, red peppers, yellow peppers, cooked green peppers, string beans, some fish, figs, dates, most melon, stews, braises, gelatinous desserts, things with heads, rabbit, veal, dill, black licorice, tarragon, lemongrass, coleslaw, mozzarella cheese, mayonnaise, rice pudding, some leafy greens, cooked cherries, fruit-flavored chocolate, peas and carrots in fried rice, tapioca, cream sauces, and anything wrapped in grape leaves or seaweed "a lot"?

Hmm, maybe it doesn't look like much when compared to those who eat only white foods.

As I continue to click my way through the online survey, I find that many of the questions don't apply to me—I haven't experienced weight fluctuation or had my eating affect my job performance, which is a good thing, since eating is *part* of my job performance—so I am thrilled to get to a question that asks me about certain textures that still bug me. Bonus: They even provide a box where I can go on at length (great length, actually, since there doesn't appear to be anything close to a character limit) about the snotty, phlegmified, baby food textures I despise to this day. The things that I've learned to categorize as "texture violations."

A few years ago, a bunch of us food bloggers were sitting around talking shop—i.e., about food. Big surprise, right? However, this time, instead of engaging in multiple foodgasms over the newest ingredient appearing on menus everywhere, we were talking about the foods we either hated or used to hate. My own whispered confession was that I couldn't stand an entire category of what I call "hot cereals." For those of you who didn't grow up standing at dark bus stops through twentysome Minnesota winters, hot cereals include things like oatmeal, cream of wheat, and Malt-O-Meal. Eating them in the morning was supposed to keep you warm throughout the day. I'd rather take my chances with the –30° windchill. As I grew up, became worldly, and experienced a variety of cuisines, polenta and grits found their way to the list along with certain desserts.[1] Because of their jiggly, slithery, snot-like consistency, tapioca, rice pudding, panna cotta, flan, and crème caramel are all access denied where my mouth is concerned.

"Oh, sure—that's a texture violation," my friend Fatemeh added matter-of-factly. The rest of the group nodded, understanding exactly what was meant. Texture violation! I finally had a term—and a relatively simple and self-explanatory one at that—with which I could tag a slew of my still-hated foods.

---

1. For the record, I will eat polenta, but only when it's grilled and firm and preferably slathered with some sort of blue cheese and mushroom sauce.

Furthermore, saying "That's a texture violation" sounds so much more sophisticated than "That's icky," like a clinical diagnosis that also comes with a hefty fine for the person who tries to make me eat a red pepper panna cotta with lemon-grass tapioca. (The fine being, of course, that I will vomit it all over said person.) Texture violation also explains why the freakishly human-like skin of peaches made them my most hated fruit for twentysome years.

On the whole, there's hardly a food word out there that disgusts me as much as "skin." I don't care how jazzed George Costanza was with his invention of pudding skins, I can't watch that *Seinfeld* episode without actively repressing a full-body gag. The first time I noted hot milk skin bringing a strange stillness to the pan was also the last time I willingly sucked down milk at any temperature other than refrigerated. Crossing off yet another task on her Big Sister Checklist, my sister wrinkled up the opaque white film with one finger and followed me around the house, trying to make me eat it. I now take my Swiss Miss with hot water.

That experience led to my phase of despising anything—fruit, vegetable, animal, mineral—with a skin. Eventually, I relented and allowed some fruits back into my life, but not the peach. I had grown far too suspicious of the fruit whose skin was distressingly similar in texture to the flesh underneath. I even preferred plums to peaches, which was confusing to some people until I argued my case:

FACT: The warmed skin of a purple plum might be the soft and pliable sort, but it seeks to maintain its own identity, distinct from the juicy, tawny depths it encases.

FACT: When you touch a plum, you do not confuse it with any part of the human body.

FACT: A plum intended for consumption is never fuzzy.

FACT: Plums do not render their flavor pernicious by staging a Fruit Cup Coup.

In my house growing up, dinner salads were often replaced with fruit alternatives: applesauce (fine, but it had to be dashed with cinnamon), Jell-O with fruit (acceptance was totally dependent on what fruit was suspended in the mass of green, red, or orange), fruit salad (usually a summer alternative, ingredients varied, therefore so did pickiness), canned pears (not bad, not great), and fruit cup (almost universally reviled).

Libby's fruit cup, which could have just as easily been Dole, depending on your time zone, was probably supposed to have a nice range of fruit. However, the only fruit I cared about was the disturbingly red maraschino cherry. My sister cared about this fruit, too. Deeply. So highly did we rate this particular component of the fruit cup, in fact, that we refused to eat our portion if the maraschino cherry was absent. Deciding this wasn't an argument she wanted to have, my mom would have to dig around in the wet depths of the fruit cup can in order to unearth two maraschino cherries. (Preferably of equal size and thickness, since she would have *heard it* if one of us got what was deemed to be "more cherry" than the other.)

The rest of the fruit cup consisted of fruits I deemed fair

to disgusting. There were white, slightly mealy pieces of pear swimming around in the preservative syrup, and while not sought after, they were benign enough to be consumed without much complaint. A second species of fruit was largely unidentifiable, and it only recently occurred to me that the stringy cubes must have been some idea of pineapple. That the stringy cubes didn't carry the actual flavor of pineapple is not their fault and, in fact, brings us to the worst fruit of all in the fruit cup: the peach.

Slippery and slimy, the peach chunks did more damage than simply violate the tongue and teeth of the texture sensitive among us. Their very flavor invaded all other flavors, surging across the borders of pear and pineapple and bullying them into peach-soaked submission. In the face of such strong-flavored oppression, the preternaturally toughened maraschino cherry was the only fruit that didn't lose its core identity.

Because of the Fruit Cup Coup, I hated everything peach flavored and refused to sink my teeth into the furry hide of a fresh peach until I was twenty-seven.

After meticulously detailing my peach hatred and explaining all my other texture violations in the box provided, I come to the section of the online Food F.A.D. survey that appears to be addressing deeper psychological issues, such as anxiety and perfectionist tendencies. There are banks of questions about the need to repeat tasks, and other questions surrounding body image, so it's clear that the researchers are casting their research net wide and considering the possibility that picky eating could be connected to other conditions such as obsessive-compulsive disorder (OCD) or anorexia.

Combining picky eating and OCD summons up the nervous image of Adrian Monk, the brilliant sad sack of a television detective who was obsessed with the number 10 and right angles, and was so riddled with phobias and anxieties that he could barely leave the house. Monk once admitted to having 312 phobias, some of which were food phobias, like his fear of milk (lactophobia) and mushrooms (mycophobia), and the fact that he had to have chicken potpie on Tuesdays. When he discovered a genetically engineered square tomato, Monk was on cloud ten, because he could finally make "the perfect sandwich," all right angles. Monk also insisted he could "taste the symmetry" and predicted that the square tomato would "virtually eliminate indigestion."

People might laugh or roll their eyes that Monk has more issues than the *National Inquirer*, but a picky eater gets Monk. He just wanted his food the way he wanted it. I call that the *When Harry Met Sally* syndrome.

This OCD section of the Food F.A.D. survey is also where the questions don't ask about food and where the instructions plead, *"Work quickly and do not think too long about the exact meaning of the question."* Which, seriously? Nice try, Survey.

I don't worry unduly about contamination if I touch an animal.

Let's see: I live with two cats who frequently get dirty cat litter trapped between their claws and paw pads. These are the same cats who sleep on my bed and sometimes even under my covers, and sometimes I find kitty litter in my sheets in the morning, which means I am, essentially spending my nights in a dirty litter box. So . . . no?

Hanging and folding my clothes at night does not take up a lot of time.

Those nights when the floor of my bedroom serves as my closet and dresser drawers? No, it does not take a lot of time to "hang" or "fold" my clothes. However, on the nights where I finally have to deal with a two-week-old pile of clothes, yes, that does take up a lot of time.

I frequently have to check things (e.g., gas or water taps, doors, etc.) several times.

See now, Survey, we ran into this problem with "a lot." You need to define "frequently." Because before I go to bed, I do check the front door to make sure it's locked. And I might check it more than once, especially if I can't remember if I locked it or checked it. (Or if I suspect that the lock has decided to unlock itself.) Same goes for my curling iron. If I don't have a very specific memory of unplugging it or seeing the cord on the floor, I have been known to get off the bus, go back home, and check. But that's because I have a history of leaving it plugged in, and it's not my aim to burn down the entire apartment building just to get my Veronica Lake wave on.

Aside from those nitpicks, which just show, yet again, how much I overthink everything, one of the things I appreciate most about the online survey—aside from their desire to help adult picky eaters—are the words chosen to describe the study. Clearly, the Food F.A.D. Study is not concealing the fact that it is being conducted on picky eaters—"finicky" is right there in the title—but the gentle wording in the introductory text is still welcome: "Scientists know very little about the range of adult eating behaviors and problems. Thus, we are conducting an online survey of unusual eating habits in adults." "Unusual eating habits" sounds more respectful than "picky" or "finicky." Of course, that's not to say that the phrasing doesn't make it sound like we are curiosities in a David Attenborough nature documentary. *"And in this Minneapolis dining room we can see the unusual eating habits of the picky eater in her natural habitat. Note how she gags on her serving of succotash even when she washes the mouthful down with prodigious amounts of water. Soon we will see how she tries to feed her unwanted vegetables to the* Felis catus *crouching under the table."*

After I finish the Food F.A.D. survey, I spend a few days fixating on one question: *"Do you consider yourself a picky eater?"* Because, to be fair, I had considered myself a reformed, recovering, or cured picky eater, but having to list the foods I still hate makes me question if I really was cured. And then there was that *"I find a lot of foods disgusting"* statement. Because, seriously, what is "a lot"? I need a precise number to assure myself that I'm not still picky. What I don't expect is that in trying to wring that precise number out of people involved in the study, I will also start doubting whether I had ever been picky at all.

Given their background with eating disorders and work with picky children, the scientists behind the Food F.A.D. Study are quite familiar with a wide range of "eating quirks" in the general population. Basically, if there's a food, there's probably

also a hatred of that food. However, those who study food aversions have found that some food hatreds crop up in greater
numbers than others. For instance, one scientist tells me that
tomatoes are a commonly hated food, which is something I
had come across in my own research as well.

My friend Chi-An, who does not consider herself a picky
eater but absolutely abhors tomatoes, tells me that her tomato
hate was all about aroma. "When I was younger," she writes
in an email, "the mere smell of tomatoes on the vine, or
tomato slices on the table, made me nauseous." Another
friend, Jeff, has a complex relationship with tomatoes where
the quantity is the issue. Chunks of tomatoes, like in salsa,
are fine, but a quarter of a tomato is too much. What about
slices of tomatoes? "I won't eat them sliced," Jeff tells me. "In
fact, I just pulled one out of my hamburger and threw it out
the window on my way home this morning."

Since the tomato haters were thick on the ground, I want to
know if there are other commonly hated foods. Secretly, I am
hoping that the group will include raisins, which are disgusting
little bits of wizened chewiness that clearly came into being
only because monks were too drunk to remember to pick all
the grapes in a timely fashion. (Even worse than regular raisins
are the lumps of earwax known as golden raisins.[2])

Much to my disappointment, raisins do not come up as a
commonly hated food. Vegetables, according to the Food

---

2. Golden raisins hide out in what appears to be a blessedly raisin-free oatmeal cookie, and when you realize belatedly that your oatmeal cookie has
been compromised, you then have to break the cookie apart and tweeze out
the golden raisins. Oh, and giving golden raisins an exotic name like "sul-
tana" doesn't endear them to me at all, *United Kingdom*.

F.A.D. scientists, and meats are widely eschewed by picky eaters. Even pasta, which some picky eaters rely heavily on, is known to nauseate other picky eaters. The strangest thing I hear from one scientist was a food *like* a lot of picky eaters share. French fries, apparently, are a friend to everyone, even the picky. Again, my own form of research backs this up, because as I search far and wide for fellow finickers, I have yet to come across one who told me they hated potatoes. I have found people who hate sweet potatoes and yams (including, until very recently, myself), but neither of those orange-fleshed vegetables counts because they aren't botanically related to plain old white potatoes, whose very plainness might be their appeal.

Potatoes are calming, soothing, and because of their bland simplicity, they don't challenge the eater with flavor too large. Potatoes are the ultimate in comfort food. In one of my most cherished cookbooks, which is based on the *Friends* television show, there's a recipe called Mashed Potatoes for the Broken Hearted, which notes, "These fluffy, smooth potatoes (with plenty of sour cream and butter) have been known to mend even the most fractured heart." In her 1983 novel *Heartburn*, Nora Ephron wrote, "Nothing like mashed potatoes when you're feeling blue" and then proceeds to give a perfectly heavenly recipe for mashed potatoes that includes the directive, "1 tablespoon heavy cream and as much melted butter and salt and pepper as you feel like." One could argue that we love potatoes so much because they are merely a vehicle for butter, cream, salt, etc., but it turns out there's a lot more going on in that complex brain of ours.

Judith Wurtman, a biochemist at MIT, has studied and written extensively about how food can influence our moods.

In *The Serotonin Power Diet*, Wurtman explains that eating carbohydrates—like our friend, the pile of mashed potatoes flooded with melted butter—causes the amino acid tryptophan to travel through the bloodstream to the brain. Once tryptophan arrives at its destination, it is converted into serotonin, a neurotransmitter that regulates mood, appetite, and sleep. If you are feeling out of sorts or down without reaching clinical levels of depression, your serotonin levels might be out of whack and in need of the boost you get from eating a steaming bowl of potatoes.

I'm also a big believer in the power of suggestion where picky eating is concerned. Just as one bad experience with a food can turn you off of it for life, repeated good experiences with a food turn you into the fan club president. It might be the placebo effect, but if a baked potato—which took you close to thirty minutes of careful stirring, tasting, and adjusting to achieve the perfect balance of butter, salt, sour cream, and sliced scallions—snagged you out of your Mean Reds on one night, you might turn to it again the next time you're feeling lousy. It's the same with picky eaters: If one food went down quietly and discreetly without causing any undue drama, you'll mentally note it as a "safe" food and even seek it out the next time you don't want to retch at the dinner table.

The same scientist who tells me about picky eaters' shared affinity for french fries also tells me that most picky eaters like bacon. Even the ones who shudder away from all other meat—be it cow, lamb, or chicken—like bacon.

My friend Lora is one of those people. At least, she's a vegetarian who makes an annual exception for bacon, even while knowing that her digestive system, having only a passing familiarity with meat, can't deal with it. She knows that her stomach, as she put it, "is going to want to remove itself from my body and run away." But she does it anyway. Why? "Because I'm craving it, I miss it, it smells like heaven, and then I'd just be miserable for two days," Lora explains.

Behold, the power of bacon. Dr. Johan Lundstrom, a scientist at Monell Chemical Senses Center who examines how the brain deals with sensory information, was sourced in a National Public Radio online article about how bacon is a "gateway meat" for vegetarians. Dr. Lundstrom told NPR, "Because bacon is one- to two-thirds fat and also has lots of protein, it speaks to our evolutionary quest for calories." Since the NPR piece was specifically addressing vegetarians, I email Dr. Lundstrom to ask if his hypothesis could be applied to picky eaters who gravitate toward bacon even if they can't stand other meat. Dr. Lundstrom replied that while he's not a feeding expert, he does believe that "the same mechanisms are at play for picky eaters." He goes on, "My understanding is that few picky eaters have aversions towards junk food (and I kind of put bacon in this category). That is because our brain is wired to like these types of food that [are] high in vital nutritional sources. One good example is actually french fries. Here you have a food source that is high not only in fast carbohydrates but also high in fat. Add some ketchup to the mix and you also have tons of sweet—all the things that the brain is wired to love and our brain is thought to store."

It's that "high in vital nutritional sources" bit that I don't want to let go of. And not just because I can conveniently trot it out to people who yell too loudly about the impurities and calories of bacon. (Just so you know, Dr. Lundstrom does note that it's not high fat or high carb intake alone that, as he delicately puts it, "contributes the most to the increase in waist measurement." It's the combo of the two that will make your bathroom scale clutch its pearls and faint dead away.) If your body isn't getting all it needs in terms of a well-balanced diet, it makes sense that your body might come to the conclusion that you are starving it, and since your body no longer trusts you to make intelligent decisions where foods are concerned, it decides to make a beeline for these things that a very smart scientist said are "high in vital nutritional sources" or that which "speaks to our evolutionary quest for calories."

Done discussing tomatoes, french fries, and bacon, I finally ask one of the Food F.A.D. scientists what their definition of "a lot" is as it pertains to the online survey statement "I find a lot of foods disgusting," the overall Food F.A.D. Study, and my picky eating identity crisis. "I don't know that we know," she admits, and explains that the online questionnaire was compiled based on existing literature on picky children, as well as information from people who have told them what their food problems were. As I write this, the Food F.A.D. Study is in the very beginning stages of research, and the current survey is meant only as a first step to learn more.

Fine, as a group, they don't know what "a lot" means, so I press this scientist to tell me what her personal definition of "a lot" would be. She explains that, to her, "a lot" would mean being unable to eat entire food groups or hating so many foods that it becomes difficult to eat in a restaurant or someone else's house.

One thing I've learned in my picky eating research is that no scientist ever wants to make absolute statements about anything. Results, facts, or theories are always assiduously accompanied by "seems," "appears," and "might." This particular scientist is no slouch in this department either, because she makes sure to note that while the above is her definition of "a lot," the science community doesn't know enough about the problem to define it yet. Right now, the Food F.A.D. Study is trying to gather information from a group of self-selected picky adults in order to find out at what point their pickiness interferes with their health and well-being.

My present-day list of disliked foods doesn't interfere with eating in restaurants or at friends' houses, so that convinces me that I definitely am a recovered picky eater. However, it is when I start to share details of my *extremely* picky childhood that the scientist brings me up short. After I list the small amount of foods I would eat, she interjects, "Right now, you are already describing a repertoire that is broader than some folks." Oh. "For the most part, you've coped just fine," she adds. It starts to filter down that I am being told that it's possible I was *never* a picky eater.

I brush that uncomfortable idea aside and try to impress her with how I got over picky eating all by myself. I explain how having good manners turned me into a lover of okra. "That's certainly interesting," she observes politely. I charge ahead and detail how I made up my mind one day to like a particularly reviled vegetable. I breathlessly tell her how I put out a call on my blog for readers to send recipes that would make me love this particularly reviled vegetable, but how I wouldn't accept anything cheese-drenched. No, I insisted on recipes that would bring out the purest character of—drum roll—disgusting, stinky Brussels sprouts! "Oh, they can be very good!" she enthuses.

Desperately, I move on to telling her about being so into food and eating that I went to culinary school, determined to expose myself to an even larger number of scary foods.

Me! A picky eater! Going to culinary school! That gets a reaction. "I want to put a bug in your ear about the fact that, as someone who understands the experience of being a relatively picky eater, one has to allow for the possibility that some folks have a more severe variant than you, and they can't just will themselves to get over it," she requests gently, and that's when she points out that I had only a "moderate problem" with picky eating. It wasn't a "disorder" for me. Explaining that there isn't a universally accepted definition of "disorder," she tells me, "But certainly there has to be distress and/or dysfunction." I leap on the word "distress" and trip over my own words to relate a terribly sad story from my childhood when I was shamed into eating my squash. I was certainly in *distress*, and the experience has kept me hating squash to this day, which is seen as a *dysfunction* by some in my acquaintance. "I understand," comes the calm, motherly voice across the phone, "but I'm not even sure that's so far out."

After I hang up the phone and pull my Dictaphone earpiece out of my itchy ear, I feel decidedly deflated. But like any rational person who has been given a diagnosis that makes them want to throw a grand mal tantrum, kicks and all, I seek a second opinion. However, when I connect with Dr. Nancy Zucker of Duke University, another big brain involved with the Food F.A.D. Study, I firmly remind myself that it is important to look beyond my preoccupation with my own food issues and continue to amass information that might help other, non-"moderate," adult picky eaters.

A specific aspect of the conversation I had with former picky eater Amy Watts really sticks with me. Amy told me that her still-picky brother is so tormented by his in-laws about his food issues that he's actually thought about putting himself through hypnosis to depickify himself. I don't have any idea if that would work, but it makes me wonder whether anyone has developed therapies for adults in the same way that they have for children. Children have long been the focus of picky eating research because picky eating can slow their growth, which can, in turn, affect their development, but adults are clearly suffering, too. And it's not just the mental anguish either. If you're eating from only one food group, eventually your health is going to suffer. In fact, Amy explained to me that part of her own impetus to get on the road to recovery was her health. "Because I was turning thirty and [I knew] that if I want to keep living, it would probably be a good idea to start eating vegetables." That sort of reasoning worked to get Amy eating more foods she didn't eat before, but other adults, her brother included, need more than that.

The goal of the Food F.A.D. Study is for the science and medical community to gain more understanding about adult picky eating so it can be defined and investigated, which will eventually help therapists and physicians develop strategies to help sufferers improve their quality of life. That's the goal, but it's a long-range goal, so I ask Dr. Zucker what adult picky eaters like Amy's brother can do right now.

"The first thing is education," Dr. Zucker says, her voice warm with emotion after I told her about Amy's brother. "The first step for him is for people to understand him. If they'd understand that obviously he didn't choose [to be picky]. It's his biology that makes things that taste pleasant to us aversive to him, and he's struggling with it. His life would be infinitely better if people left him the hell alone." I interrupt Dr. Zucker to verify that picky eaters aren't just struggling with taste, but that textures of food can be offensive, too. "Absolutely,"

Dr. Zucker responds. "His quality of life would increase exponentially if everyone who cared about him tried to understand a little more about what his experience was and stop trying to change him!" Dr. Zucker goes on, without missing a beat, while I do a mini-jig around my living room at the vehemence in her voice. Finally, speaking directly to the brother's in-laws, Dr. Zucker concludes, "So let's all stop pushing and allow him to just experience that you guys 'get' him first."

Out of breath from my mini-jig, I flop back down on the couch and yet again bring up my biggest problem with the Food F.A.D. Study: What the heck do you Food F.A.D. people mean by "a lot"? Dr. Zucker gives a laughing sigh and explains that the current questionnaire is only their first attempt and she admits they need to rework it, adding she knows it's a subjective question. "My experience with picky eaters: You know if you are one," Dr. Zucker concludes. I confess to Dr. Zucker that the more I learn about picky eating in its increasingly severe forms, the less sure I am about whether or not I was really a picky eater. "To me, if your fear of eating new foods got at all in the way of your functioning, then I would say, yeah, it's relevant," Dr. Zucker says. So, once again, I tell my harrowing childhood squash story.

The acorn squash in front of me was cold and orange. And squishy and maple-syruped and gross. I didn't want to eat it. I couldn't eat it. My mom made some things I didn't like—zucchini, spinach, succotash, and string beans being the worst of the group—but she never, ever made me eat orange squash. But this mother was making me eat it. In fact, this mother was making me sit alone in her cold, long dining room until I finished the seeping pile of mush in front of me.

When my mother baked cookies, she let us eat the leftover cookie dough. (Salmonella wasn't a screaming headline back in those days.) This mother didn't allow her kids to eat the leftover cookie dough. This mother took any remaining cookie dough—be it sugar cookie, chocolate chip, oatmeal, or peanut butter—and added it to the leftover dough she was accumulating in the freezer. When she had enough dough to make a single cookie, she made it and she baked it off. This mother's kids were never allowed to eat dough scraps. This mother's kids were also not allowed to just have three bites, and be done with a food that had no business being put in front of them ever.

Squash.

Aside from Jell-O, no food was more aptly named/has lived up to its name more.

Squash.

Squish.

Mush.

Squaaaaaaaash. Ish.

I was sitting at this mother's table with this mother's squash in front of me because I was staying with a neighborhood friend—her kid—while my parents were out of town. After she had announced to the family—her husband and two kids—that "Stephanie will be sitting here until she finishes, everyone else can be excused," the dining room had cleared out. We were engaged in a battle of wills. I wasn't being stubborn; I knew for a fact that if I ate the entirety of the wet orange mess that I would gag it all up. You might think that would have taught her a lesson, but you'd be wrong. She was the kind of person who would have accused me of throwing it up on purpose.

Somehow—using a complex method of swallow, gag, swallow again, wait, get a new bite—I got it all down. I don't remember how, but I do remember that I knew I had to finish it so I could get away from that cold table and that cold room and that cold mother. The sooner I ate it, the sooner I could go to bed, and the sooner my parents would come and take me back home, where I was never made to clean my plate.

Was that traumatic enough? I ask Dr. Zucker. Can I still claim I was a picky eater? I hold my breath, waiting for her to validate my picky identity. "Oh, there's no question," Dr. Zucker reassures me. "If you were afraid of eating at friends' houses, that puts you in a different category." I quickly explain that as a kid I also had a multitiered system of avoiding food at the dinner table. "All these things—it interfering with attention, interfering with functioning—all these things take it away from just being a little selective, in my opinion," Dr. Zucker adds.

Even after years of research spawned by the Food F.A.D. Study, what exactly makes a picky eater a picky eater might always be difficult to define. Clearly, from one perspective, I wasn't a picky eater as a kid because the sheer number of foods I hated wasn't extensive enough. Another perspective would call me picky even today simply because I hate raisins. "You know if you are one," is what Dr. Zucker said. So from where the director of the Duke Center for Eating Disorders sat, I could stop worrying about whether I was a former picky eater. Instead, I could start worrying about whether I was *raising* a picky eater.

CHAPTER 5

Are You a Hypomomdriac?

In this day and age, one of the things you do as new and expectant parents is get the pee scared out of you at infant safety classes. A few years ago, I was at such a class where we were told about outlet covers, cabinet locks, oven locks, toilet locks, and doorknob cages. We were instructed to get rid of all glass coffee tables, rubberize every sharp edge in the house, and how scaring the baby to tears by screaming "DANGER! DANGER!" would be a really good way to teach him a safety lesson about playing in the litter box.

I was rolling my eyes at the infant safety gear catalogs being passed around the room until the instructor asked if we knew how to use our fire extinguishers. Suddenly, I flashed on all the fire extinguisher gags in sitcoms and wondered, "Wait, do I?" Next thought: "How do you try out a fire extinguisher without using all of it? Is that even possible?" Then the instructor went on about removing the plastic ring and how it might be tricky. "WHAT PLASTIC RING?! OH GOD, I HAVE TO GO HOME RIGHT NOW AND PUT OUT A

FAKE FIRE AND THEN BUY ANOTHER FIRE EXTIN-
GUISHER!"

Somehow, Mark clearly sensed where my silent panic was taking me. He muttered out of the corner of his mouth, "Merit badge in fire safety." My breath whooshed out. It's good to be married to an Eagle Scout. Especially when you are teetering on the edge of parenthood and freaking out about every little thing.

Except eating. While I might have been a picky child and adult, and while I am the kind of person who finds it extremely worrisome when I've run out of things to worry about, I wasn't worried about my baby's eating. In fact, after my experience chatting with kindergarteners in San Francisco, I have good reason to believe that picky children are becoming scarce.

Interviewing the five-year-old set was supposed to be an easy way to harvest a bunch of funny quotes from the age group I thought I could rely on not only to be picky but also to be vocal about it. It would be sort of a "Kids Say the Darnedest Things: The Picky Eater Edition." After asking a few friends with school-age kids how to go about visiting classrooms of children that weren't my own, I get linked up with a kindergarten teacher in San Francisco who invites me up to the city.

As instructed by my contact on the teaching staff, I hang around the frigid play yard at the elementary school in Bernal Heights and try really hard not to feel like a child molester until the classes come screaming outside for recess. While the kids sit in a large circle and snack on oranges, the teacher introduces me in both English and Spanish. "Stephanie is a writer! She's writing a book! Her book is about food! She wants to talk to you about food!" Talking to kids requires a lot of exclamation points. It can be especially helpful when you're trying to get them to do something they don't want to do.

"Henry! We're going to take a nap! We're going to see teddy! We're going to be cozy!" The teacher explains to the kids that if they want to talk to me about food, I will be sitting near the main door. With thirty pairs of eyes fixed on me, I walk self-consciously over to my assigned bench with my Tupperware box of food and hope one or two kids will want to chat.

I turn when I hear a roar of little feet pounding after me. They swarm me. Three crawl up on either side of me. Five line up behind my back. Four more close off escape routes directly to my left and right. I am horribly reminded of that scene from *Suddenly Last Summer* when the village boys surround Sebastian. I just hope the kids aren't *that* kind of hungry. I mean, how much can oranges really fill you up?

Now that I have the kids' attention, I figure it will be easy to get them to dish on the food they hate. I could not be more wrong. These kids actually like, nay, *love* broccoli and Brussels sprouts. One child tells me she is "mad" when her mom doesn't have Brussels sprouts for dinner. In vain I ask, "What are the yucky foods?" and I get back, "I have to say, there isn't anything I don't like," "I like the flavors of broccoli," and "I love Brussels [sprouts]. If someone gave me one, I'd stuff it in my mouth." (This is accompanied by a demonstration of said mouth stuffing.) Finally, one kid admits, "I don't like beans because they are brown" and another chimes in, "My least favorite thing is lox." But it takes a lot of prodding to get even those small crumbs. On the drive back home, I shake my head. Five-year-olds aren't supposed to love Brussels sprouts and broccoli! What's wrong with kids today?

There are several factors that might explain this phenomenon, but it all comes down to an early exposure to a wider variety of food than what existed thirty years ago. The number of ethnic restaurants and markets in urban areas has increased, which means children have more opportunities to try foods that might not appear on their kitchen table or in the school lunchroom. Sure, I loved Vietnamese and Chinese food as a kid, but I hadn't even heard of the Persian or Afghani dishes I love now and offer to my own son. Add to that the proliferation of local farmers' markets over the past ten or so years, and you have kids eating fresh, in-season vegetables, which are so much tastier than out-of-season produce and worlds better than the frozen and canned varieties kids of the seventies and eighties grew up eating. Even jarred baby food has gotten exotic! Not to take this train down the "when I was a kid, I walked barefoot to school in the snow, uphill both ways" track, but back in the seventies, aside from a few weird flavors ("beef w/ beef heart," anyone?), Gerber's baby food combos were pretty pedestrian. Especially by the standards of today, when parents find themselves popping open a jar to feed their babies something called Chicken Mango Risotto for dinner.

Outside the home, some restaurants are catering to or encouraging sophisticated palates in the preschool set by overhauling their children's menus to include items such as grilled Arctic char and roasted pork loin and nixing the comforting grilled cheese staple. Even plain and nonthreatening macaroni and cheese has been reinvented with fresh pasta, peas, and Parmesan (a rendition that would have made me cry as a child). It seems natural that an urban exposure to a wider variety of food—restaurants, home cooking, and the jarred stuff—is the reason why those San Francisco kindergarteners are evidence of a disturbing new breed of *un*picky eaters.

Kids have gotten so sophisticated that gourmet cooking camps are springing up all over the country to fill a need.

Instead of making lanyards and ceramic ashtrays, these budding foodies are spending their summers learning how to braise, sauté, and grow shiitake mushrooms on a log. At Chef Kelly Q. Dietrich's Kids Culinary Summer Camp of Vermont, kids between the ages of ten and seventeen milk cows and make cheese, decorate cakes, learn how to garden and raise fish, explore ethnic cuisines (South American and Japanese, to name a few), and take culinary field trips to places like cider mills and trout hatcheries. There's even a four-week-long "Intensive Culinary Camp" for kids who are interested in pursuing careers in the culinary arts. As for what the kids can expect to eat while at the Kids Culinary Summer Camp of Vermont, it's not the typical cafeteria-style food found at most camps. An article profiling the camp in the *Wall Street Journal* notes that counselors do "light cooking" for the campers, but that "most meals are made up of the campers' own creations."

It's undoubtedly wonderful to have that sort of variety in summer activities, but it also makes me wonder if we expect all kids to become little adults with gourmet palates at too young an age. That's fine for those who do have those palates, but not so fine for the kids who don't, the drawback being that with the increase of mini-gourmets also comes an increase of food acceptance expectations on the part of parents. See, it used to be that kids like me were tagged as picky eaters when we didn't eat our vegetables, but I'm beginning to wonder if these days some kids are being called picky if they're grossed out by stuff like seaweed and offal. Yet even with the growth of these culinary camps and hearing proud parents brag about their kids requesting pork belly and sushi on a regular basis—stuff I had never heard of as a kid and probably wouldn't have touched even if I had—picky kids still bedevil their parents.

Soon after my experience with the Brussels sprouts–loving kindergarteners, I come across a post on a parenting bulletin board requesting input on a feeding clinic. (That's another thing you do as new parents: join parenting bulletin boards. Where else would you learn about nursery schools, read reactions to wipe warmers, or find advice on how to get your kid to stop gnawing on the furniture?) I might be all grown up and capable of deciding that it's perfectly acceptable for me to breakfast on ice-cream sandwiches, but learning that something called a "feeding clinic" exists for picky eaters brings on sweaty hallucinations of being packed off to said clinic because I wouldn't eat my string beans. Has picky eating really become such a thorn in the side of parents that feeding clinics have cropped up to deal with it? And what sort of reprogramming goes on in such places? Would they have taken me on as a patient because, after a minor choking incident, I once faked a fear of steak to get out of eating it? Like a responsible writer, I set about arranging a visit to the clinic to get my questions answered.

I blame the classic movie diet on which my mother fed my nascent pop culture appetite for inspiring fantasies that I'd only be taken to the clinic's "showrooms," where everything was nice and clean and sane and, you know, not like *Snake Pit* at all. Yet I would *know* that behind other closed doors they chained children to tables and forced them to watch *Veggie Tales* and *Big Night* over and over again. Unfortunately, citing concerns about the privacy of their clients, the clinic I contact declines all requests, wheedles, and begs for an interview. Since I can't glean anything about their cost or methods from their strangely opaque website, I try *hard* to change their minds. I tell them I don't need to see or meet any of their clients. I tell them we can conduct an interview over the phone and I won't even set foot in the clinic. I just want to know what they do for picky eaters and if they would have taken on eight-year-old me as a client. But it's to no avail. I can't even get this clinic to tell me if their methods are similar to the pediatric feeding disorders program at the Maryland-based Kennedy Krieger Institute, which takes an "interdisciplinary team approach" that brings in nutritionists, gastroenterologists, occupational therapists, behavioral psychologists, social workers, and speech pathologists.

For the briefest of moments, I entertain the idea of getting my intel by nefarious and wholly unethical means. I could use my baby as a prop and pretend that I am seeking help for him. But that would be wrong. Instead, I'll use my baby as a prop at the playground! (Which seems less wrong. Probably because of the swings.) I start viewing the other playground parents as potential sources. I'll use my son's plump cheeks and masses of dark hair to lure innocent parents to my side. One look into his round blue eyes and they'll fold like a bad simile about stuff that folds.

But I restrain myself.

Instead, I go back to the online bulletin board, where one mother offers to tell me about her experience at the same feeding clinic that stonewalled me.

When her daughter was a year old, Sarah, who doesn't recall being a picky eater herself, struggled to get her to eat more than just a few flavors of pureed baby foods. After a few months, concerns surrounding Sarah's daughter's health and weight arose, so she consulted with her pediatrician and a nutritionist, and got a referral for the feeding clinic. After her initial interview at the clinic, where her daughter's eating habits were assessed, Sarah was told she could have her child treated at the clinic or she could try the clinic's feeding methods at home.

At the clinic her daughter would be strapped into a chair (much like a regular high chair, despite the disturbing images the word "strapped" conjures) until she finished whatever food she was given. "They basically said, 'It doesn't matter if she screams, cries, vomits, she's gotta finish it,'" Sarah tells me over the phone, adding that she did think the feeding clinic's methods were "severe." However, Sarah explains that the children are *not* force-fed. No one at the clinic prizes open their mouths with a rubber-tipped spoon and packs the food in. The spoon is simply held in front of the baby's mouth and not removed until the baby takes a bite. It's a form of behavior modification that doesn't allow the baby to use various methods, like crying or swatting the food away, to refuse the food. Essentially, the baby learns that the spoon does not go away until the baby eats the food.

Instead of schlepping her daughter to the clinic several times a day for this treatment, Sarah decided she would try the feeding clinic's method at home. As it turned out, that was no picnic for anyone either. Sarah's daughter spit out the food, cried, kicked, and screamed, and after a few weeks, Sarah stopped. She realized that it wasn't worth all the hassle and decided to give her daughter more time to develop better eating habits. Sarah adds, "It's not just that it's disgusting, but you really feel like you're hurting your child."

Meanwhile, the whole experience did teach Sarah's daughter the importance of eating and that finishing what was in front of her meant she could get out of the high chair. Sarah continued to encourage her daughter to try more things. Today, Sarah calls her daughter a "moderate eater." She doesn't eat everything, but she's much better than she used to be. She especially likes her grandmother's food, which is due in some part to the fun names Sarah's mother gave to the food. Calling bits of stir-fried chicken "chicken nuk nuk" would make Sarah's daughter pause, look at the food, and then try it rather than refusing it outright.

That exact picky eating ploy is the plot of Lauren Child's children's book *I Will Never Not Ever Eat a Tomato*, in which a boy gets his picky little sister to eat by giving the food fantastical names. I shove that little trick up my sleeve, because my research is having the unfortunate side effect of convincing me that Henry is coming down with a case of picky eating.

You see, I'm a hypomomdriac. Hypomomdria, a special neurosis experienced by parents, manifests itself when the subject learns about a phase, a problem, or a disease and automatically assumes it's going to happen to their kid.[1] I can't even read the emails from various parenting websites anymore, because when their newsletter headlines say things like, "Is your baby really happy?" my knee-jerk reaction is, "I don't know—is he? Wait, are they asking if he is *too* happy or if he's *truly* happy? And which one is bad? Which one means autism?" (That's another thing I've learned as a parent: Practically every single thing your child does can be a sign of autism. Possibly. Maybe.)

At 5 pounds, 10 ounces, Henry wasn't technically underweight when he was born, but his size did mean we had to wake him up to eat (smaller babies often sleep through their hunger pang wake-up call) and keep track of how many

---

1. And with that, I've just blessed the world with another fantastically annoying word. You also have me to thank for "cheftestant."

ounces he was consuming at each feeding. When he turned a year old, we were long past the point of hauling out the roasting pan and kitchen scale to obsessively weigh him between checkups, and our pediatrician was more than happy with his weight. But having been so concerned about every ounce that went into his body since day one, I am finding it a little difficult to stop worrying, especially now that he is starting to refuse various purees. Though it is apparently commonplace (read: normal) for a kid to reject a food fifteen to twenty times before finally accepting it, once I learn that picky eating could be a sign of something called sensory processing disorder, guess what diagnosis Dr. Hypomomdria comes up with?

Sensory processing disorder (SPD) is a neurological disorder in which the affected individuals are overly sensitive to various sensory stimuli. It could be that fire engine sirens are significantly louder and far more disturbing to an SPD sufferer than to others, or that the feel of certain fabrics against their skin squicks them out. (Hmm, Henry has suddenly started acting as if the glistening drifts of bubbles in his bath are trying to attack him whenever they touch any part of his body . . . more fuel on my hypomomdria fire!) Occupational therapists are often called upon to try and help alleviate the condition. When dealing with auditory or tactile issues, for instance, the occupational therapy might include listening to custom-made music and sounds or being touched with special skin brushes to help the brain learn how to desensitize the stimuli and deal with it in a calmer manner. If SPD-based sensitivity extends to the sufferer's mouth and tongue, the texture and temperature of certain foods can be repellant to them and that leads to picky eating.

Unfortunately for parents dealing with SPD, not all doctors recognize it as an actual disorder. Sensory issues are not fully understood at this time, and the current lack of comprehensive research means that insurance companies won't foot the bill for needed therapies. "It's a terrible thing to be a human being and have a problem that affects you or your child and to have some doctor tell you it's *not* a problem, and even if it were a problem, no one's going to pay for treatment. That's terrible," one of the Duke Food F.A.D. scientists tells me when we discuss SPD and picky eating.

My friend Joyce Slaton, a food writer who has recently written a number of articles on picky eating, has a five-year-old daughter who was diagnosed with SPD. In her first year, Joyce's daughter, Violet, ate everything, and Joyce, who is like me—a former picky eater turned foodie—admits that she was over the moon about it.

"'She likes it! She likes it!' I crowed about my organic, salt-free, lightly steamed spinach. My husband and I clung together, thrilled at the miracle of a baby eating spinach. Surely we were the best parents who ever lived," Joyce wrote in a Babycenter.com post called "My picky eater stole my smug." But then things changed. Violet hit the magical mystical age of eighteen months—supposedly a time when so much changes for baby and parents—and she went picky on Joyce. Gone was the baby who opened her mouth for chicken vindaloo and Swiss chard risotto; Violet now eats no meat and no vegetables.

At home in Violet's presence, Joyce is loudly demonstrative about how much she loves her vegetables, hoping that Violet will respond with what scientists call "modeling" and want to copy her mom's enthusiasm for vegetables.

However, the Monkey See, Monkey Do approach doesn't always work, and one thing Joyce has learned in her own picky eating research is that the more a parent directly pushes a child to try a disliked/disfavored food against their will, the more they will resist. As the scientists in a 1998 *Appetite* journal article put it, "It has been consistently shown that parental pressure to consume foods is associated with higher expression of food neophobia" and "future presentations of the food will be associated with the parents' exasperations and the child will continue to reject the food."

In other words, "Lay off, Mom and Dad, you're just making it worse." Another manifestation of this quintessentially childhood phenomenon happens when parents try to decrabbify kids by addressing said crabbiness head-on. When my mom singsonged, "*Someone* woke up on the wrong side of the bed todaaaay!" she was trying to jolly us out of our moods, but the fact of the matter was she just bought herself a couple more hours of sullenness. That's how perverse kids are.

Recent research indicates that breastfeeding might help prevent picky eating. Whatever the mom eats, the baby eats via breast milk, which means a greater exposure to a variety of flavors they wouldn't get if they were formula-fed. However, Violet is one example of how breastfeeding won't defray pickiness, at least not when SPD is involved. How long did Joyce breastfeed? "Three and a half years!" Joyce shrieks down the phone to me. "That kid ate everything I did!"

But Joyce powers through, employing other methods to get Violet interested in vegetables. "I have *sewn* her vegetables out of felt, we have *grown* vegetables in gardens, we have painted still lifes of vegetables, I mean, I have done every goddamned thing you can imagine," Joyce tells me, her voice rising with incredulity. "I have Violet watch *Veggie Tales* in hopes that she'll enjoy veggies—that's actually one of my therapies. Of course, she's getting Christianized at the same time," she adds with a burst of her throaty laugh. Even after all this, Violet's veggie interest hasn't piqued yet, but Joyce won't stop trying. She also won't get too amped up about it. Joyce with her bright sheaf of Hubba Bubba pink hair is not someone you would ever call uptight or anxious. "I model healthy eating. I talk about how great my vegetable dishes are. And I hope," she calmly wrote in a blog post.

It's really too bad that Joyce's calm, Zen-like approach doesn't filter through my thick skull, because my anxiety over Henry's potential picky eating and SPD reaches "OH MY GOD, WHAT IF I HAVE TO SEND HIM TO THE FEEDING CLINIC?" levels the night I attend a picky children lecture arranged by a local parenting group.[2] Although my initial intention was to be an observer, a note taker, and to practically study the other parents around me like bugs under a glass, I find myself dragged into my own experiment.

Given its proximity to San Francisco and Silicon Valley, the town of Belmont is bewilderingly woodsy. A few blocks off El Camino, which is sort of a mini-highway in the Bay Area, I take a wrong turn and hit a dead end. As I flip the Prius into a U-turn, I am startled to see that my silent car has surprised a family of deer poking around a residential alley.

---

2. FACT: The more anxious and cautious among us are the ones who are more likely to be afraid of trying new foods. Scientists have concluded that "sensation seeking" types are less likely to have food neophobia. If you are a skydiving, roller-coaster-riding, bungee-jumping sort of adrenaline junkie, chances are lower that you're a picky eater.

I lock eyes with the mother while her two younglings scramble away and then, trying to make myself seem as unthreatening as possible, I noiselessly slide the car back down the street and find my way to the senior center where the lecture is being held. Once out of my car, I feel as if I'm in two worlds. I can hear the traffic on El Camino, but over my head sweep monolithic redwoods, and drifts of pine needles scritch under my shoes. I stand outside and inhale the camp smell—a mixture of pine sap and log buildings gone slightly mildewed—willing myself to go inside and work.

Inside, rows of metal folding chairs are set up in an echoing, high-ceilinged rec room, where remnants of a craft sale are also in evidence. The incoming crowd of parents that pick their way around tables strewn with pinecone ornaments and cellophane bags of squashed homemade cookies mostly consists of mothers with a few fathers sprinkled here and there.

After everyone finds a seat and examines the multicolored sheaf of healthy eating handouts on their chairs, the president of the Belmont Mom's Club introduces the speaker, Karen Ross, a registered dietician, nutritionist, and health educator. Trim and smiling with silvering bobbed hair, Karen greets us enthusiastically and gives a brief lecture about encouraging good eating habits in our children and setting goals for ourselves as parents. We then break into small groups to discuss our specific concerns. I lay out my observations for the other parents: One day Henry loves sweet potatoes, the next day he hates them. One day he eats everything put in front of him and asks for more; the next day he eats three bites the entire day. The parents around me, who are nodding their heads in agreement and sympathy, reveal they are having very similar experiences with their toddlers.

When we reconvene as a larger group, Karen listens to our various concerns and offers advice on how to combat what she says are perfectly normal eating habits for children. However, while she addresses specific situations like kids who eat too much sugar or breakfast only on cereal bars, Karen's overriding message to all of us gathered here tonight is that we really need to relax and not feel like it's the end of the world just because some kids have suddenly turned into carbivores.

When I talk one-on-one to Karen in her sunny Palo Alto kitchen a few weeks later, she asks if there's a way to approach her talks in order to get through the thick neurotic skulls of my generation (my words, not hers—she is very respectful). "I find talking to parents of preschool children really compelling, I also find it really frustrating. It's my most frustrating audience. What am I *not* saying?" Karen wonders, bemused.

I explain my personal hypomomdria and how it's practically impossible for my generation to take the laid-back approach to parenting. We always feel like we're falling down on the job or we're not doing enough to perfect the lives of our adorable pieces of progeny. Oh, and that every empty box on the pediatrician's developmental checklist is clearly our fault.

Given to you at various pediatrician visits, the developmental checklist (aka the "What isn't your kid doing yet?" checklist) fills most parents with dread. Some parents get the checklist in advance of their next visit, so they can actually work on the next expected developmental milestones, but others spend their time in the waiting room getting unnecessarily worked up and defensive. (And by "others," I mean "me and my husband.") Not wanting the other parents to know what our son is or isn't doing, Mark and I sit in the waiting room and whisper-shout things like, "He doesn't know his body parts—we haven't even *tried* to teach him his body parts yet! Wait, but he knows 'truck,' 'ball,' 'kitty,' and 'bottle'—can I write that instead?" and "Okay, well, he *does* talk! I mean, he says things, but they're in his language, not human language, is that what they're asking?!"

"Yeah, I don't think you all are as relaxed," Karen notes dryly and adds, "I never focused on [picky eating] at all, and I don't know any of my friends that focused on it." Were her two children picky at all? She takes a sip of coffee as she considers this for a moment before she says thoughtfully, "You know, my husband said they were." She continues, "I didn't pay any attention to whether or not they liked green beans, or whatever. I took the attitude of: I served what I wanted to serve, and that was it."

In other words, Karen avoided doing what pediatric feeding expert and author Ellyn Satter calls "short-order cooking." And short-order cooking is exactly what I have been doing with Henry. When I offer Henry food that he refuses or doesn't eat enough of to satisfy me, I dash about the kitchen, opening more baby food jars or pulling stuff out of the fridge that I know he would like. Why? Because he needs to eat, doesn't he? He has to eat *something*!

Satter warns against the short-order cooking approach for various reasons. In the first place, it allows your child to believe you will always be this accommodating, which, let's face it, is impossible, and it doesn't teach them discipline or boundaries. It teaches them that with a little bit of whining, their parents will always cater to their whims and caprices. Second, constantly making alternative meals will drive you nuts and wear you out. (Tip: When you find yourself swirling water around the coffee carafe to pour yourself a cup of caffeinated water, you might be worn out.) Instead, Satter advises offering a variety of choices at mealtime, including one thing you know your kid will eat. If they eat all or some, great. If they eat nothing, fine. Walk away and let it go. (It should go without saying that the "walk away and let it go" approach should not be used when your kid's weight and health are in jeopardy, but I'm going to say it anyway.) And since she acknowledges that a kid might refuse a new food (vegetables, usually) fifteen to twenty times before they voluntarily eat it, she advises parents to be persistent but neutral when offering these foods. They'll try it someday.

Another very important point both Karen and Satter make is to avoid the clean-your-plate rubric, the three-bites-and-you're-done rule, and even the just-take-ONE-bite-*please* mind-set. While forcing any of these methods might make the parents feel better that their child is eating enough and well, it teaches the kids to override their own internal sense of fullness or satiety. It's also a sign, Satter says, that the parent is being overly controlling. And not to get all doom-and-gloom about it, but forcing a kid to eat past their satiety limits like that could lead to issues of either obesity or eating disorders later in life.

Keeping mealtimes pleasant and relaxed is another one of Satter's recommendations. While difficult mealtimes are hard on the parents, they are harder on the child, who easily picks up on the tension around him. If meals keep turning into fights over what isn't being eaten, the child has the potential to go through life feeling that food is just one big steaming pile of stress and become an increasingly picky eater as a result. If you want to look at it purely from a physiological—rather than psychological—standpoint, stress can wreak havoc on the entire digestive process, resulting in lack of appetite, nausea, cramping, and acid reflux. Yum! Meanwhile, if mealtimes are presented as a calm and happy time when everyone is together, enjoying one another as well as the food in front of them, it can help children associate food and eating with pleasant and good feelings. (See Chapter 6 for more on emotions and eating.)

A genial dining atmosphere can really make all the difference to a picky eater. We hear all the time how making sure to sit down to family meals with your kids can improve their lives in so many ways—staying out of gangs, off drugs, in school, etc.—it makes me wonder if the influence of the family table is the reason why my husband became such a food lover and why Anderson Cooper takes very little pleasure from food.

On his daytime talk show, Anderson confessed to eating a very limited range of foods. He even said that if he could drink every meal in the form of a protein shake, he would. However, Anderson, who devoted an entire episode to his distaste of most food, including hot beverages, cannot blame his pickiness on being a supertaster. He proved that when he, along with his audience, took the paper taste test challenge and he tasted nothing. Not even the slightest bitterness that I, the average taster, can detect.[3] Based on that reaction, Anderson seems to be more like my husband: an undertaster. But unlike my food-loving husband, who may not taste all

---

3. Of course, I feel obliged to remind you that Dr. Reed doesn't put a whole lot of faith in those paper taste tests.

the subtleties food has to offer and whose penchant for adding hot sauce and pepper flakes to everything speaks to a need to punch up food to a higher level of flavor that his palate can detect, Anderson does not derive any enjoyment from food. He is annoyed that we have to eat and sees it merely as fuel. Eating is just something that has to be done and there's no getting around it.

What makes Anderson Cooper the undertaster so different from my husband, who is also an undertaster but eats everything? Aside from Anderson relating that the family joke in his house was that they had two courses in their household—Aquavit and Carr's table water crackers for pâté—I can't pretend to know the intimate details of his mealtimes, but I know that in my husband's house, food was very much enjoyed and discussed at length by the entire family. And they didn't just talk about how the food tasted, they talked about how everything was cooked, how it was prepped for cooking, what the individual ingredients were, and where they came from. In every possible way, food was enjoyed to its fullest.

At the end of their frayed rope, it's easy to see why parents seek the help of a feeding clinic, as Sarah did, but others, like Joyce, might go to an occupational therapist. When it comes to feeding issues, occupational therapy deals with the physical movements of the mouth, whereas cognitive-based therapies take a stab at changing or adapting existing behaviors or reactions. Some feeding specialists, such as Dr. Nancy Zucker, who does cognitive behavioral therapy at the Duke Center for Eating Disorders, believe that a good picky eating program should include an occupational therapist. Dr. Zucker tells me that pediatric feeding clinics are recommended for babies and children who have "functional impairments" or other medical problems that get in the way of eating. She would not have recommended that a picky eater like me be sent to a feeding clinic. "Because you have the luxury of having a lot more time when health is not immediately impaired," Dr. Zucker explains. "If your kid is not getting enough nutrition to survive, the stakes are much higher." In that sort of situation, the child is diagnosed as "failure to thrive."

While the current definition of "failure to thrive" (FTT) applies to a baby or child who weighs significantly less than they should at their stage of development, Marianna Thorn, the inpatient therapy supervisor of the occupational therapy department at Lucile-Packard's Children's Hospital, tells me that the diagnosis has a very *Jane Eyre*-ian past. Initially, it was specifically applied to children who weren't being cared for or loved enough. These children weren't held. They weren't touched. And the lack of such affection was detrimental to their growth and development. Bunny Crumpacker offers a chilling description of failure to thrive in *The Sex Life of Food*: "[The babies] are deprived of the simplest ingredients of the love they need: familiarity, cuddling, trust. Such babies may refuse to eat, or they eat too little to prosper. Their hunger strike has severe consequences. They become listless and withdrawn; they don't grow properly. Their motor skills develop poorly and late. Sometimes they don't learn to speak. Sometimes they don't survive."

Marianna works with babies and school-age kids who are FTT, and she also sees children whose weight and general nutrition are fine, but whose family still has concerns surrounding the eating/feeding process and need advice on how to handle meals. However, when picky toddlers are brought into the hospital that sits on the palm tree–packed Stanford campus, Marianna warns parents that picky eating at this stage is simply a normal developmental phase.

In their early years, starting at one and extending into age six, kids are pushing for more control and independence than ever before. At a year old, babies are no longer blobs of drooling softness, who need parents to do everything for them. Toddlers are walking, running, caterwauling windup toys, who never appear to need a battery change and who want to do everything themselves. Adding to the potentially picky scenario is the size of a toddler's stomach: it's small and it fills up quickly. These little ones know when they're full, even if we don't believe they could have possibly eaten enough to make it through the day. A frustrated friend posted on Facebook about her sixteen-month-old's eating issues, and one of the responses was, "Toddlers seem to live on air and love." It's almost a disservice to tag kids as picky at this age, because it is so typical and normal.

"We see [toddlers]," Marianna tells me as we sit in one of the physical therapy rooms at the hospital. "But there aren't going to be a lot of changes, because we are doing everything against what they want to do." Additionally, because their sensory awareness is naturally heightened at this age, Marianna explains that it's quite common for a toddler to be more bothered by things they are hearing, touching, or tasting than they ever were before. (Ah, Henry's fear of bubbles: normal, not SPD.) Because of this, instead of wiping the baby down after every pureed bite, Marianna wants parents to let their babies get messy at the table. It helps accustom them to the feel of food on their hands, and counteracts the "ICK!" factor they might feel when touching their food. Marianna reasons that if a child is grossed out by the feel of food on his hands, he probably isn't going to allow that food in his mouth. "And that could play a role—even in a child without feeding problems—in making them more picky," Marianna tells me.

A way that parents can nudge the desensitization process along is to make sure their babies experience a variety of food textures as early as possible. An article on MSNBC.com suggested that parents today feed their babies the smooth purees longer than necessary, and that babies actually have the ability to deal with more textures earlier than we think. Marianna explains that parents stick with smooth purees for an extended period of time because if a baby gags on purees at six months of age, it's likely that the pediatrician will say the baby isn't ready for the purees and suggest waiting a bit. However, this "waiting a bit" goes on and on until, suddenly, the baby is ten months old, and she's still eating only the very smooth stuff when she should be experiencing and adapting to new textures. "So instead of going through the desensitization part of it, [the parents] try to go around it, or they stay behind it and [the kids] never desensitize," Marianna concludes.

An additional benefit babies reap from eating textured foods is the development of their oral motor skills. As the food goes from smooth purees to textured purees and finally finger food, the baby's mouth is getting more physically involved in the eating process. By chewing and using their tongues to manipulate and move pieces of food around their mouths, they are gaining strength in their tongue and jaw. If this necessary strength doesn't develop properly, the child will have problems with voluntary swallowing, they might not be able to hold their mouths closed, and they will encounter issues with speech development. Before my visit to Lucile-Packard's, if I ever really thought of it at all, I thought of speech as something that developed by listening to and imitating those around you. I never even considered the physical needs required to make talking happen. Eating builds language.

As an occupational therapist, Marianna helps babies and children whose oral and tactile sensitivities are getting in the way of their eating/feeding process. Some of them also have hyperactive (easily triggered) gag reflexes, which might be due to their heightened sensitivity or because they had a bad experience with solid food early on. This "bad experience," known as a learned experience or one-trial learning, only has to happen once for it to adversely affect the baby or child's association with food.

Whether we're picky eaters or not, we've all had at least one "learned experience" with food in our lives. Mostly, it's when we eat something and later get to experience the delights of having our systems rewind and forcibly eject it like a bad videotape. It doesn't matter if it was the food or something else that made you blow chunks, because now the food and vomiting are too inextricably entwined for you to want to eat—or be anywhere near—that food again for a long time, if ever. Your brain, body, and senses have now *learned* that particular food equals vomiting and become averse to it out of self-preservation. Because I once got carsick while chewing Trident spearmint gum, I can't abide the flavor of spearmint. Even though I know that the gum isn't what caused my car sickness, my self-preservation instinct is so strong that it overrules my intellectual reasoning and will always connect the taste and smell of spearmint with nausea.

You don't even have to take it all the way to vomiting to create a negative impact; just gagging on a food is enough to scare children off eating certain foods or textures. Marianna tells me about kids who are so scared of eating that they gag when just a spoon is put in front of them, or even when the refrigerator door opens. In one situation, a child was presented with a teething biscuit and he gagged at the sight of it, so Marianna left it on his tray. However, simply being able to see the biscuit got him so upset that he began to shake and cry.

When I ask Marianna if she thinks childhood picky eating is on the decline at all, she shakes her head. "I definitely think it's on the increase," she told me. I tell Marianna of my experience with the Brussels sprouts–loving kindergarteners and posit that maybe it just seems like picky eating is on the increase because our culinary standards have been elevated in a world where sushi and pork belly have become as commonplace as fish sticks and pork chops. Marianna mulls this over and says, "Either that, or we're just more aware of it now. I bet if you asked your mother [about your picky eating], she probably didn't obsess over it." (She definitely didn't.) From what Marianna's seen, today's parents are so fixated on obesity and heart disease that they are cutting back on fat and calories in their children's diets at a time when children actually need fat and calories to grow and develop properly. "And this is really terrible to say," Marianna continues, "but I think—being more educated—that older parents are more focused on those things."

Of course she's right. A 2011 article in the *New York Times* quoted Andrew J. Cherlin, a demographer from Johns Hopkins, stating that college-educated women are waiting until they finish college and start a career before they get married and make the move into motherhood. This is a trend, the article noted, that "accelerated" in the 1980s. A few days later, citing the *New York Times* article, a *Psychology Today* writer published a piece on egg freezing and fertility, which came to the conclusion that "more and more women are having babies after the age of 35."

Since I had my son when I was thirty-five, I am part of that trend, and for us older parents, those extra years of waiting to have kids come with sackloads of time to get older and wiser. And by "wiser," I mean "collect all the information out there to make sure we are sufficiently freaked out by every stage of parenting." We have instant, Google-propelled access to too much information, and it's overwhelming and paralyzing at times. We have TV news, newspapers, magazines, blogs, and email newsletters. And we talk. We talk a lot. And I say "we" because I know I'm not the only mother out there like this.

There's the mother in my circle who won't use a white noise machine to help her baby sleep because she read somewhere that it might do long-term damage to his hearing. And there's another one I call my Facebook Eeyore because every time I say anything on Facebook about my pregnancy or new motherhood, she dooms-and-glooms all over it. When I commented that pregnancy did to my stick-straight hair what years of Ogilvy perm burns couldn't, she said, "Just wait until the postpartum hair loss." I looked forward to a prenatal massage, and she warned, "Make sure you clear any massage with your doctor!" I mentioned Henry had his first cough, and she wrote, "Hopefully it's not the croup!" I'm a neurotic, sure, but I'm not the only one. Just saying.

After my son was born, I learned pretty quickly that I couldn't be judgmental of other parents and their decisions.

Before he came along, oh, man, I could judge with the best of them! Is that your kid whining in the checkout line? Well, why did you bring him if he can't behave in public? Be quiet, screaming baby on the plane, don't you know that all of us annoyed adults were perfect flyers as babies? But now, I can't help putting myself in other parents' shoes. If I see a baby or a child doing something that raises eyebrows or draws glares, I have nothing but empathy for how that parent feels.

I'm no longer capable of judging any parent for the decisions they have to make for the health and welfare of their family.[4] And that includes needing the services of an occupational therapist or a feeding clinic or deciding on another course of action entirely. It's not one-size-fits-all when it comes to picky children. I might follow Satter's advice about "no short-order cooking" with Henry, but that never would have worked with my friend Julie Burba. Her aversions were so physically intense that her mother actually did have to make Julie different food from the rest of the family or Julie simply would have been unable to eat. Now, as a grown-up, she loves food. Not only did Julie go to culinary school, but she's also an event chef and the director of marketing and communications at that culinary school. Just like with adults, there are myriad reasons why children might be averse to certain foods and just as many potential "fixes" or preventatives that can be attempted, but there isn't one answer to the "How can I fix my picky kid?" question. It's good for parents of the non-

---

4. Within reason, of course. If you tell me you let your kid smoke two packs of cigarettes a day like that baby in Sumatra, I'm probably going to judge you. By the way, that baby has finally kicked his habit.

picky to remember that, too. Whatever you did—or didn't do—to ensure you have a "good" eater, keep in mind that it's not necessarily going to work for another family.

For my part in this saga of hypomomdria, as much as I disturbed myself with my research and imagined all sorts of worst-case scenarios for Henry, I have since calmed down and stopped worrying about his eating. Just like Joyce does for Violet, I give Henry a variety of foods, and he eats happily and very well on some days and less well on other days. He still has plenty of time to go picky on me, but I'm not so freaked out by that prospect as I once was. The great thing about having too much information at my neurotic fingertips is that I have a better idea of my options if Henry's eating really goes downhill. I still don't know what path I'd choose, but at least I know there are paths.

CHAPTER 6

The Picky Eater's Emotional Stomach

Put your hand on your stomach.

I'm serious. Put your hand on your stomach.

I'll wait.

Did you do it? Next, think of eating the most disgusting food you can imagine . . .

Got it in your mind?

Okay, now make an "ew, gross" face.

Did you feel your stomach clench?

Congratulations, you've just completed your first lesson in how emotions affect digestion! Now, since that was also your *only* lesson in how emotions affect digestion, let's review: Hand on stomach, icky food thought, stomach reacts by clenching.

Why? Well, according to Dr. Zucker, who walks me through the stomach-clench test during our interview, anxiety—such as the anxiety picky eaters experience when they sit down at the dreaded dinner table to eat a dreaded plate of black spinach seeping dreaded ichor all over the plate—messes with your digestion. When you're extremely anxious, your body kicks its fight-or-flight response into gear, just as if a tiger were in the room. (That's right, being made to eat a food you don't like is as scary as having a tiger crouched over there by your green recycling bin. Just ask any picky eater.)

"What your body does," Dr. Zucker tells me, "is go through all these changes to facilitate your escape. [Your body decides], 'We don't have time to digest food right now. Digesting food takes a lot of energy, and we cannot expend that energy on digesting food, we gotta get you the hell outta here!'" So instead of processing what you just ate, your body forces food to sit in a lump in your stomach—it's called "delayed gastric emptying"—which will make you both uncomfortable and nauseous.

By the way, for those of you who didn't pass the stomach-clench test, don't feel bad. Mark couldn't manage it either, even though I instructed him to imagine eating apples with slices of cheddar and stacks of bologna sandwiches. (Those are the only foods he hates so much that, as I write this, he is in the kitchen, covering his ears, singing, "LALALALA—I'M NOT LISTENING TO WHAT YOU ARE TYPING!")

"Maybe it only happens to picky eaters?" Mark wonders after his stomach-clench failure and then pauses. "Wait—it happens when I think of *Gilmore Girls*. Does that count?"

Thinking about stress and eating is actually something I've been doing since fifth grade, when one of my teachers told us that stress at mealtimes made the stomach turn red and messed up digestion. Armed with that knowledge, I became a tyrannical little hall monitor at our family dinner table, and whenever conversations got . . . difficult, I'd remind everyone why they should cut out all the yelling. "MY STOM-

ACH IS TURNING RED!" was also my response when my parents tried to discuss grades at the dinner table. Since they still make fun of me for this, I suspect my parents believe I completely made it up. Dr. Zucker, what do you say?

Dr. Zucker laughs that she can't confirm the color your stomach turns in such a situation, but she agrees that keeping mealtimes as free from anxiety as possible helps everyone's digestion, not just that of a picky eater. Helping a picky eater manage mealtime anxieties, however, is not as simple as putting a cork in "Why wasn't that B-plus an A-minus?" discussions. When she works with picky eater kids, Dr. Zucker has a three-step approach that can also be applied to adults.

The first step is convincing the picky eater that their food issues are not character flaws or something to be ashamed of; they're simply part of who they are.

Starting with the biological explanation, we all remember Mr. Rogers praising individuality when he sang, "There's only one in this wonderful world, you are special," right? Every one of us is biologically wired in a way that makes us unique, even from our family members. We hear differently, we see differently, we feel differently, and most important, we *taste* differently. That's all a function of having discrete biology. However, the biological explanation is not one people associate with picky eating. "Understanding different people's tastes is something that people struggle with a great deal, because you can't get your mind around what it tastes like for them," Dr. Zucker says. "Because you aren't living in their mouth, so you can't possibly understand what they're experiencing," I add. "Exactly," Dr. Zucker confirms. "We can understand someone else's sadness because we've felt sad."

Alternately, a picky eater might hate chicken because they

had a particularly negative encounter with it at some point. This is part of the picky eater's "learning history." Referring to her method of treating picky eaters, Dr. Zucker details, "We explore their learning history, so that they can really validate why they are the way they are [and] that it makes perfect sense, given what they've experienced, that this is the range of food they're willing to have." Rather than feeling that they are to blame for disliking so many foods, picky eaters could either shrug their picky eating off as part of their biology (genes, taste receptors, etc.) or they could point to their learning history (bad chicken experience = chicken avoidance). In either case, it's not their fault and it's not their choice.

In this first step, when the picky eater accepts that she isn't to blame for her food choices, she can stop wasting energy running a defense game with everyone who questions her food choices and is able to concentrate on moving forward to accepting more food into her life. "It's amazing what can happen once someone has been understood—how it frees one up to shift," Dr. Zucker concludes.

Dr. Zucker's second step concentrates on changing the negative association of mealtime. Picky eaters dread meals in advance, and once your mind—that powerful little coil of sloshing gray matter—has decided that something is going to suck, your body will respond in kind by shutting itself off to food (the aforementioned fight-or-flight response), and the battle is over before the first course even hits the table. Dr. Zucker deals with this by explaining to family members exactly what is going on with the picky eater and getting them to make mealtimes more enjoyable and less of a place where the picky eater feels the need to fend off the rampaging broccoli forest. "Even if nothing changes in terms of the content of food," Dr. Zucker elaborates, she encourages the families to see mealtimes as a time "when we break bread together, we share our days together, and it becomes this beautiful, sacred time where the family comes together."

The final step of Dr. Zucker's process is where the actual eating comes in, but before the food hits the mouth, Dr. Zucker tries to get picky eaters to relax their bodies by using progressive muscle relaxation (PMR). This technique, which is also used to combat other physical complaints like restless leg syndrome, insomnia, and anxiety attacks, starts with the leg muscles. Eyes closed, the person tenses the leg muscles for about ten seconds and relaxes for twenty seconds, before moving on to the muscles in the abdomen, chest, arms, and face. Dr. Zucker's personal picky twist to PMR is to get her picky eaters to make "playful disgust faces" and then relax out of them, mindfully unclenching jaws and facial muscles. This process, which is sure to elicit giggles, would also seem to take the wind right out of the "ew, gross" face's sails, sort of akin to how Hogwarts students in the Harry Potter novels are instructed to deal with malevolent shape-shifting boggarts by changing the boggart into something silly and then laughing it away.[1]

Once they're relaxed, Dr. Zucker invites her picky eaters to really get to know the food in front of them. First, the picky eaters examine the food intently and describe what they see using only neutral words. Sticking to neutral words, those

---

1. And did you know that because laughter is such a great way to destress, you can actually take laughing yoga classes? I just hope that the laughter is real—like the instructor is really good at stand-up—and not a forced "Laughing Hour" as in *Star Trek: The Next Generation*.

that describe color, shape, size, and texture, is very important. The picky eaters can't say the food is "gross" or "delicious," because the point is to avoid prejudging the food, which could set off the undesired chain of stomach events: clenching (potential reddening) and refusing food's entry. The same descriptive process is undertaken when the picky eaters are told to sniff their food.

Not to get Miss Manners-ly all of a sudden, but I was always taught that sniffing one's food was considered very rude. Granted, when my sister and I did this to my mom's food, the sniff was immediately followed by dramatic gags and nose scrunching, but isn't that just because we didn't properly relax our bodies as prescribed by Dr. Zucker's second step? Let's look at some etiquette evidence:

In *At Home*, Bill Bryson notes that in the nineteenth century, "It was not polite in refined circles to smell a piece of meat while it was on one's fork." He doesn't explain why, but it does beg the obvious follow-up questions: "What if said piece of meat resided on one's plate, prithee, kind sir?" or "What if, pray tell, 'tweren't meat but 'twas vegetable that my fork presented?" (Now, the nineteenth century was also when a man dropped trou in the dining room and peed in a bucket that was stored in the polished mahogany sideboard specifically for such a purpose, and no one said boo about it, so consider that as well.) Moving on to a more contemporary source, the Peace Corps' website has a fascinating section called "Cultural Gaffes at Home and Abroad." Here you can learn all sorts of imperative international Don'ts, including which direction to face your butt at a concert or play in Denmark. The list also includes the information that sniffing at your plate in Uganda would suggest to your hosts that you suspect your food is spoiled. Very uncool thing for a guest to do.

Okay, fine, so my sister and I were rude on two different continents as well as in the past. However, I see no reason to interrupt Dr. Zucker with this information as she goes on to tell me what happens after her picky eaters have sniffed and described their food. If they're up for it, Dr. Zucker explains, the picky eaters take a bite of the food and describe what they taste, again using neutral words.

The whole point of Dr. Zucker's food examination and description exercises is to make picky eaters so curious about the food in front of them that their hate for it is dialed down to a level where it becomes background noise. "By observing and perceiving, they're also lowering their arousal," Dr. Zucker goes on. In other words, because they're looking at the food in a new way and seeing it in a new, neutral context, they aren't so fixated on how gross it is, which might make them a little more receptive to eating it. Dr. Zucker elaborates, "The more we think, the more our emotions are being regulated." And emotions don't just reside in the stomach and body of a picky eater either. Oh no, my friend, sometimes they get cooked *right into your food*.

"If you cook with love, people will love what you cook!" I was quoting Jacques Pépin from my flopped position on the couch. My entire hand was covered in dried blood from a paring knife incident, and I was way too tired (or weak from the blood loss) to think up my own words. It was my first week working in KQED's back kitchen on the set of Jacques Pépin's cooking show *More Fast Food My Way*, and I knew I had hit on a picky eating epiphany. Jacques was saying that if you love to cook so much that you care deeply about the process, you're going to make good food that everyone loves. Which reminded me of how much my mom *doesn't* like to cook.

In her own words, my mom is "an indifferent cook." To her, cooking is a tiresome chore.[2] Now that I'm all grown up, I can finally comprehend that making meals for her persnickety (and sometimes ungracious) family was a huge pain in the ass, which is why I'm not going to get into that long line of whiny writers who blame their mothers for everything wrong in their life. I can't blame Mom for putting cooking on par with cleaning toilets any more than you could blame me for liking the color blue. It's simply a preference, and she simply doesn't enjoy cooking.[3] However, Jacques's quote—and a subsequent shallow dip into Hare Krishna beliefs—got me gnawing at the idea that Mom's "indifference" in the kitchen may have affected how I felt about the food.

If she saw cooking as a chore, maybe I saw eating it as a chore. Instead of it being a time where we all relished one another's company, as Dr. Zucker would wish, maybe the whole dining environment felt like drudgery on some level. I ask Dr. Zucker what role (if any) she thinks the parental enjoyment of cooking plays in picky eating. "I think it has a

---

2. That's why it didn't go over real well when my dad gave her a Cuisinart for Christmas. Because giving a kitchen appliance to the woman who dissected frogs and earthworms in her spare time was no different from giving her a vacuum cleaner. Sort of, "Hey, here's a chore you can do with an extra-sharp blade!" Mom wanted an electron microscope, not something that pulsed out pestos.

3. And really, how *could* she enjoy cooking for a family who energetically greeted her breaded veal experiment with lolling tongues, gagging, and my dad saying, "We've never had *this* before. How . . . interesting. Is it supposed to be that color?"

huge impact," she tells me. "Picking up on these subtle, non-verbal cues that cooking is a drag, that eating is a drag, probably makes someone a little more thoughtful about it or a little more hesitant."

One could argue that there's an amount of carelessness brought to the entire cooking process when you don't derive any pleasure from it. You follow the recipes and directions, sure, but you don't dig any deeper. You don't taste as you go—checking the dish for optimal seasoning and flavor balance—and you don't spend time learning more about food or experimenting with recipes, which, among other things, would teach you the best methods to cook certain foods. Like how roasting Brussels sprouts instead of steaming them makes worlds of difference in terms of flavor. Because if cooking is a chore for you, why would you spend any more time than absolutely necessary on it? It would be like researching various toilet-cleaning methods for fun, which no one but the Monica Gellers among us would want to do. When it's a chore, cooking, like cleaning toilets, is a "get in and get out" kind of deal.

Again, I'm not blaming my mom. She had three kids, three cats, my dad, and a house to take care of. Trying to force interest where there was none would have been a pointless waste of time when one daughter is sitting screaming in the bathtub with lipstick all over her face, the other is trying to make toast in the microwave,[4] the oldest is stealing her dad's pajamas to make into skirts, the cats are peeing in various

---

4. Yeah, that was me. I burned two holes in my parents' brand-new microwave.

corners in the house, and Dad is aimlessly shuffling around the kitchen wondering, "When's dinner going to be ready?"

However, the meals I loved most also happened to be made up of my mother's favorite foods. Maybe her own love of those foods meant she enjoyed cooking them and took the time to do them right. For instance, my mom loves lamb, and I always requested lamb chops for my birthday dinner. Not that they were served at my birthday *party*, mind you, which was a time for cake, ice cream, and frozen stacks of Totino's pizzas, but lamb chops were what I asked my mom to make when we had the family birthday dinner and they were always perfect.

In discussing this theory, my friend Rachel points out that lamb chops are a really weird thing for a picky eater to like. As are, she goes on, two other of my favorite foods: artichokes and escargot. Granted, but with artichokes, you have the winning combination of getting to play with your food—usually a dinnertime no-no—paired up with a ramekin of melted butter. I put it to you that it is impossible to dislike a food when you get to pull it to pieces with your fingers, dip parts of it in a hot, golden pool of butter, and toss the rest of it aside. And it's not that artichokes don't taste amazing, because they do, but even if they didn't, your teeth don't scrape off enough artichoke to be offensive in the face of all that butter.

This brings up the obvious question: "Wait—but you ate *snails*! How can you call yourself a *picky eater*?" This is how: fat man in a red suit. My family had escargot once a year as part of our traditional Christmas Eve dinner of appetizers (or "tidbits," in my family's parlance) and we ate them sitting cross-legged on the floor. The whole atmosphere—from eating off the coffee table to our meal being lit only by a lively fire and a sparkling Christmas tree—crackled with excitement and anticipation. BAM! Right there you've got your "beautiful, sacred time where the family comes together," as prescribed by Dr. Zucker.

Furthermore, my parents never forced us to try the snails my mother had so lovingly stuffed into bake-able shells and buried under mounds of green snail butter.[5] There was no cajoling, no fighting, no battlefield scarred with the oozing remains of succotash and zucchini, just an open invitation to try the snails if we felt like it. Recalling what Ellyn Satter said about getting kids to eat, every meal should be like eating escargot. The food you put on the table for your kids is an open invitation. There should be no pressure to taste, and no forcing if any part of the meal is declined. Plus, eating escargot was yet another way to play with my food. I grabbed up the hot snail shells with special pincers and then used special teeny-tiny forks to prick out the tender nuggets of butter-basted meat. If we turned our noses up at our portion of snails, my parents were more than happy to eat our share as well. I'm sure that their pure enjoyment of the escargot went a long way to encourage us to partake of the Christmas treat.

So, I liked the foods my mother liked, either because she took more care cooking those foods than she did with others or because I was modeling—being strongly influenced by my parents' behavior and reaction to things. Or it was a combination of the two. And in the reverse, I didn't like the foods she didn't care as much about. (Although in the interest of

---

5. Snail butter is green because of the minced parsley.

full disclosure, I should say that I didn't like *all* the foods she loved, because she loved liver and onions and there was no way I was touching that plate of hot sick.) Granted, I've heard plenty of stories of foodie parents who love to cook and still end up with picky kids, but it's one possible explanation for my experience.

The other way I could use my mom's dislike of cooking as a picky eating scapegoat is if I fervently believed Mom wasn't just adding V8 juice and pepper, but that she was literally mixing her emotions into her meatloaf.[6] Which would mean I converted to Hare Krishna.

Anyway, so there I was, muttering, "If you cook with love, people will love your food." (Which actually came out as, "Eef you cooook weeth luff, peeepol will luff your foooood," not because of blood loss but because I was trying to speak in a French accent.) Well, that spawned an outburst from Mark:

"Wait, that's like that thing! From *This American Life*? You know, there was that guy who dated a girl and she said that she had to break up with the guy because he had to meet chefs to make sure they weren't angry when they cooked his food. Remember? That *thing*!"

I opened one eye and looked at Mark. I wasn't delirious from losing a pint of blood or from being on my feet for ten straight hours, running from kitchen to set to kitchen to set. No, it's simply that there are times when my husband plain doesn't make any sense and he gets impatient when I don't understand him.

That *thing* he was referring to was a story called "Cringe

---

6. It should go without saying that my mom's meatloaf is better than your mom's. After having my son, I had her make and freeze three loaves for us.

Crush," about a woman who dated a guy who had converted to Hare Krishna and insisted on meeting chefs/cooks before he would agree to eat in restaurants. Because they believe that animals have souls and are created by God (Krishna), the Hare Krishnas don't eat meat. But beyond that, they also believe that if you eat the product of a violent act like animal slaughter, your consciousness will absorb that violence, which could lead to you having violent thoughts and committing violent deeds. You're not just sitting down to a nice, juicy hamburger; you're sitting down to a plate of road rage. With fries.

The Hare Krishna concept of various consciousnesses using food as a conduit also extends to what goes down in the kitchen. Whatever emotions the chef is feeling get transferred into the food she makes, and whoever eats that food also eats and absorbs the emotions. ("If you cook with love, people will love your food.") To a Hare Krishna, it then makes sense to assess the cook or chef's mental status before sitting down to a meal in her restaurant. Then again, I don't know what happens if you meet the chef, determine she's happy enough to make your grilled cheese, and then unbeknownst to you she gets pissed off at the busboy while flipping your sandwich. I guess it's entirely possible that you get pissed off later in the day and don't know why.

Before I met Jacques or learned anything about the Hare Krishna religion, I already had my own parallel mantra: "Never cook angry." The longer version of that mantra is, "If you're pissed off because your *Alias* DVDs arrived scratched and unplayable from Netflix, *and* it's the weekend with no hope of getting replacement DVDs any earlier than Wednesday, you shouldn't try to bake a loaf of bread because you will end up setting your kitchen on fire." Which I did, because I somehow managed to swap parchment paper with wax paper and was richly rewarded with a flaming oven, a ruined loaf of rustic Italian bread, and the revolting stench of scorched wax paper stinking up the joint.

Never cook angry.

(I blame Netflix.)

Now, it is true that I threw out the ruined rustic Italian loaf without serving it to anyone, so I didn't actually witness any anger being transferred via toast. (Although considering that I would be serving them slices of bread that tasted like funky candles, I think it's safe to assume they would have been pissed off.) However, it is still a good example of how angry cooking leads to angry food. Bearing this in mind, I bring the topic up with Dr. Zucker, who tells me she finds the food and mood connection fascinating. "I think attention has a lot to do with it," she says. "There's a lot of literature on the role of attention and emotion, and when we're in more pleasant moods, our attention is much more expansive as well. You're willing to be more creative. When we're anxious or angry, we're focused on escape and getting done." Yes, it can be argued that my Netflix anger distracted me and made me inattentive enough to exchange parchment paper for wax, but there are also times where negative emotions alone, not negative emotions leading to inattention or carelessness, affect my cooking. Or at least my taste buds.

In times of stress, I have put together a meal that is technically perfect. And by "technically perfect," I don't mean it's going to win any challenge on *Top Chef*. What I mean is I executed the recipe to the letter. I didn't make a parchment paper-wax paper mistake. I didn't leave out ingredients or bungle amounts. It's the same dish or meal I've made and enjoyed countless other times, yet when I sit down to eat this meal I've prepared while stressed, sad, or angry, it tastes like crap to me.

However, since my sweet garbage disposal of a husband always proclaims that the meals that taste awful and unsatisfying to me still taste wonderful to him, I question the poetic and spiritual explanation I gleaned from both the Hare Krishna beliefs (sacrilege!) and my idol Jacques Pépin (snackrilege!). Mark is not tasting my stress, sadness, and anger in a meal I most certainly prepared *without* love, so if he couldn't taste what I tasted, maybe my moods are somehow seeping into my taste buds and messing with them.

Most everyone has come across the "food to ashes" metaphor so popular with authors. As in, "Upon hearing that her fiancé was marrying her just for her inheritance, Hortense's food turned to ashes in her mouth." Food to ashes references are found in the Bible, Milton, a speech by John F. Kennedy, song lyrics, and even in the movie *Pirates of the Caribbean*. The reasons for the transformative event can range from idol worship to curses, but when used as a literary device in novels, it's clear that there's something going on emotionally that causes the character's food to taste bad. Since it's such a universally accepted event, and one that I've had personal experience with, I imagine there must be some bit of science behind it.

Being a late-night TV watcher—a time when I unwillingly consume a prodigious amount of diet pill infomercials—I'm already well acquainted with the notion that stress causes your body to release the hormone cortisol, which supposedly ends up making you fat in the long run. If a mood can make you fat, can a mood make your food "turn to ashes" in your mouth?

I ask Dr. Reed at Monell if there's anything to the idea that if you're pissed off, your tongue might be, too. "Regarding the effect of mood on the taste system," Dr. Reed emails me, "taste receptor cells on the tongue contain receptors for a variety of hormones and so a reasonable case might be made for the impact of physiological changes, including mood state, to alter taste perception." Aha! If you read very carefully, you will see that Dr. Reed is saying, "Yes, if you are pissed off, your ability to taste things might be affected." Essentially. Dr. Reed adds, "But this topic has not received much experimental attention." I'm sure. Can you imagine the requirements for a study on how emotions affect taste? "Are you an angry woman over the age of thirty-five? If so, please join us in a study where you should be prepared to be annoyed, irritated, or otherwise enraged on a regular basis. Come hungry: You will be fed, but you might be too pissed off to eat."

Remember how Alexander ends his Terrible, Horrible, No Good, Very Bad Day by being served lima beans for dinner, and he *hates* lima beans? That's author Judith Viorst showing that she gets how emotional eating is. Yes, Alexander has already dragged himself through a comically train-wrecked day that featured dropping his sweater in the sink, cavities, and ugly railroad pajamas, but the fact that he has to eat something gross for dinner makes it so much worse. He can't even seek solace from dreaded kissing on television and a too-hot bath in the comforting form of crunchy Shake 'n Bake pork chops and mashed potatoes.

If I'm already bordering on a black mood, I often rely heavily on a favorite meal to yank me out of it. Sometimes it works, and I become a shiny, happy person having fun. However, if, for one reason or another, the meal is subpar, it can send me to the depths of despair. The inverse is also true. Food—really, really good, amazing food—can also make me deliriously happy, it can deliver me from evil, and it can even restore my faith in humanity. And yes, I'm aware that makes me sound like a manic-depressive.

"It's always scrambled eggs. There's something about it that's so basic and easy and comforting." After wrestling her two kids to bed and settling in for the night, my friend Joy talks to me about the food she relies on to soothe fractured nerves and prop up a flagging mood. "It's like this great big exhale. Like, I'm fed. It's going to be okay. And even if I haven't been able to shop, I know I always have eggs on hand," Joy adds. For additional comfort, Joy doesn't turn to a glass of wine to accompany her meal; she pours out a glass of chocolate milk. "Because that's from childhood," she explains.

In her book *A Natural History of the Senses*, Diane Ackerman gives one explanation why childhood foods might be associated with comfort and how this association starts very early in life. "The first thing we taste is milk from our mother's breast, accompanied by love and affection, stroking, a sense of security, warmth, and well-being, our first intense feelings of pleasure . . . such powerful associations do not fade easily, if at all." Another reason why people seek solace in the food they enjoyed as children could stem from a desire to go back— maybe not to the womb exactly—but to a time when life was simpler, when worries were fewer, and when the worries that did exist were small. It's a need to return, if only for a moment, to a time when we were looked after. It's a need for a brief respite from the present, when, as adults, we look after ourselves, in addition to others. Until the folks at NASA perfect time travel—and by the way, can we get on that, people?—replicating that cocoon of tranquillity in a bowl of mashed potatoes is the closest we can get to turning back the clock.

However, sometimes the food that soothes us, the food that you can look at and say, "See, you *get* me, food," isn't necessarily food with roots in our childhood. Quite simply, it's food that you enjoy for its flavors or its textures or its serene simplicity. In her book, *Cooking for Mr. Latte*, food writer and former *New York Times* food columnist Amanda Hesser discusses the pleasure that can be found in cooking a quiet meal for oneself. However, the impetus that drives her to the grocery store on the night she describes in her chapter "Single Cuisine" is not fueled by the sudden desire to prepare a solitary meal, but a need to relax. As she puts ingredients in her basket, Hesser notes that she is planning a meal that is "self-soothing"; it is comfort food, a meal that will smooth out ruffled nerves and a jangled mental state. Hesser then goes on to list examples of her friends' "home-alone" food—one friend stirs up polenta with white truffle oil, another makes gourmet grilled cheese sandwiches—before detailing her own favorite solitary meals. Hesser acknowledges that her solitary suppers of poached eggs on bitter greens or hard-boiled eggs sieved over asparagus are "not traditional comfort food, but it works for me." When Hesser sits down to eat her home-alone meal on this particular night (a simple green salad and toast topped with a fluff of scrambled eggs and truffle oil), she writes, "The toast calmed my nerves. I carefully ate my salad, carving the leaves into manageable pieces. I heard a door shut outside, but otherwise it was silent." Comfort. Peace. Calm. It's about treating yourself well by indulging in foods you enjoy.

My own ideal, mood-boosting comfort food has very few ingredients, all of which I keep on hand: pasta, Parmigiano-Reggiano, olive oil, sea salt, and pepper. If I have it and I feel like dragging out my knife, I might add minced parsley or chives for color and a bit of meditative chopping therapy. On the night that Mark was working late and a breached diaper had me following a trail of poop dollops down the hall to their giggling owner, I substituted butter for the olive oil, which made everything—even the post-bath, peeing-on-the-floor incident that followed the breached diaper—much, much better. Other times, like a day that starts with an entire carton of eggs smashed on the kitchen floor, ends with me stepping in cold cat vomit *in my bare feet*, and has a whole mess of crap going on in between, I recognize that it's just better for all involved to give the kitchen a wide birth and let someone else do the cooking. In our house, this means ordering out for deliciously bad Chinese food.

It wasn't always like that, though. Food wasn't something that could make or break my moods for a long time. Instead, food was often something I actively feared and dreaded. Especially when I had to go to events that featured strange food at friends' houses or even stranger food at unfamiliar restaurants. I didn't analyze my anxiety and fear at that age; Kid Me simply didn't want to eat gross food. It was basic, it was primal, and it was in my gut, which is precisely where I *didn't* want the food. Adult Me was fully cognizant of the source of my anxiety and fear. Less worried about the act of eating gross food, Adult Me was more concerned with how I would camouflage what I saw as my total lack of sophistication.

I was compelled to hide my pickiness because I was terrified of what people would think of me if they found out I was stuck in an eating never-never land, where I lived immature and stunted, surviving on corn, grilled cheese, and lamb chops.

If you haven't already come to this conclusion, being a picky eater is a perfectly wretched state to be in. And one that can be achingly lonely. Some picky eaters are so miserable and self-conscious they turn down all dining-out invitations, including the ones involving their families and holidays, rather than expose their picky eating or be made vulnerable by it. Dr. Zucker would like to get picky eaters—the adult and child variety—to an emotional place where they can own their pickiness, where they are not ashamed and are not allowing it to be a source of constant stress in their lives. She wants picky eaters to be able to say, "This isn't my fault, it's not a flaw. It's my biology and it's just the way I am," and really believe it. This level of calm, assured self-acceptance would empower picky eaters to go to restaurants and dinner parties without fearing what might be lurking in casseroles or in the minds of their friends and family.

Coming boldly and confidently out of the picky eating closet is a great goal, but it is a difficult one, too, and it's also one I never achieved. (Well, maybe not until I wrote a book announcing my pickiness to all and sundry.) Instead, as an extremely self-conscious person who worries far too much about what others think of me, my picky eating embarrass-ment (my PEE, if you will) forced me to eat foods in restau-rants and at dinner parties that I would not have otherwise touched with a ten-foot spork. While it did cause me certain anxiety, it had an unexpected side effect. It made me fall in love with foods I thought I hated.

CHAPTER 7

The Picky Eater Eats Out

"So, um, does slicing them ahead of time make them less slimy?" I asked carefully as Catherine pulled a bowl of prepped okra from her fridge. "Nope, it just saves time," she responded, skating a pat of butter across a hot skillet. Oh.

Five minutes earlier, Mark and I had arrived for dinner, and Catherine announced we were having catfish and okra. Okra? Oh, god. Oh, goddy god god. As a recovered picky eater, I had gotten to the point where I could finally handle—even enjoy—most vegetables, but okra? Who on *Mother Earth* makes okra north of the Mason-Dixon Line? My Virginia-raised friend Catherine, that's who, and I was going to have to eat it. I knew this, I accepted this, and I tried to plan for it by pretending to be completely engrossed in how the okra was being prepared.

"Butter and olive oil!" I noted, infusing my voice with marvel, while my brain chanted *Slimy okra, bad okra, evil okra, GAG!* Catherine scattered coarse salt over the sizzling green pentagons before clapping a lid over them, explaining, "I'm just going to let them steam for a bit." "Ah," I smiled, nodding knowingly. *(Green okra, seedy okra, wet okra, GAG!)*

When we sat down to dinner, Catherine passed the bowl of okra around the table. I took a small spoonful and carefully spilled it out next to my catfish. "They got a little more brown than I wanted," Catherine said apologetically as she took a bite. "Oh, I'm sure it's delicious," I said, breathing deeply to keep my gag reflex in check, as I raised my own fork to my mouth. *(SMELLY OKRA, MUSHY OKRA, CRUSTY OKRA, GAG!)*

Every picky eater—former or current—has been in this situation. And every *adult* picky eater knows that dinner parties are their personal hell. I put special stress on "adult" because when you're a picky child, the meal doesn't matter. Any meal at someone else's house is a minefield of potential gustatory explosions. Even my husband—a self-proclaimed "professional eater," who really doesn't dislike any food except bologna—recalls of his childhood, "There were some parents who didn't *understand* peanut butter and jelly sandwiches, and you just never ate lunch at their houses."

The man has a point. I'm willing to bet that every child can rattle off the neighborhood parents who never grasped the delicate jelly to peanut butter ratio, the houses where crunchy supplanted creamy, and still others who used the wrong kind of jelly or bread. In my experience, white bread was better than wheat—the sandwich should be able to be smushed and molded into an edible ball, if the eater so desired—and strawberry or grape (no seeds, chunks, or any sign of actual fruit, thanks) were really the only acceptable options for jelly. That was bad enough, but it wasn't nearly as bad as the parents who expected you to [wait for it] *clean your plate!*

Now, most parents were sympathetic to kids and food and didn't push the issue. Even my own parents expected us to eat only three bites of a food we despised, but those other parents? *Shudder.* Because I didn't dare try all the food avoidance tricks my sister and I pulled at home, the only thing I could do at the Clean Plate houses was wait it out and hope that the Clean Plate parents would eventually relent because baby-sitting my dinner plate was keeping them from watching *Hill Street Blues.*

When it came right down to it, the safest place for a picky kid was the school lunchroom. Not in eating the school lunches—because unless it was that wonderful spongy pizza, hot school lunches were pretty gross—but in eating your bagged or lunch-boxed meal. The meal your mom packed hoping you wouldn't throw it out. I wasn't allowed to pack my own lunch until my mom was reasonably assured I wouldn't claim a balanced lunch was made up of Ding Dongs (dairy!), Doritos (corn-ish!), and Fruit Roll-Ups (fruit-like!). In the school lunchroom with the bottomless gray plastic trash barrels, there were no parents checking your pockets for food-stuffed napkins, no one counting your bites. There wasn't even a plate to clean. Your lunch box went to school full, came home empty, and whatever happened to the contents between home and school was between you and the trashcans.

My parents did raise me to have good manners, and Kid Me knew that refusing to eat the food at other people's houses was bad manners. But that sensibility was heavily outweighed by just how much I didn't want to eat that food. It's as if Kid

Me hadn't quite grasped the concept of "rude." I understood "polite," because that just meant saying "please" and "thank you" at appropriate times. That it was rude of me not to eat the food eluded me until adulthood. (Frankly, I thought it was rude of them to *expect* me to eat the food when I so clearly hated it.) The one good thing about eating at a Clean Plate house was that I never made the same mistake twice. One meal was all it took and then their doorframe got marked with cherry Kool-Aid to warn all the other kids in the neighborhood to pass over that house for dinner.

As a kid, you can pretty much get away with that sort of behavior, but as an adult you are expected to know better. The idea that pickiness is one of the immature trappings of childhood you are expected to outgrow along with (public) nose picking is something that weighs heavily on a lot of picky eaters. It either causes them great anxiety at a friend's dinner party or keeps them absent from those types of functions entirely. I didn't avoid dinner parties, but they did make me very anxious for a considerable amount of time. However, in a strange reversal of fortune, those very dinner parties—combined in equal parts with the manners my parents infused into me—ended up being one of the things that helped me get past my picky eating.

Let's rewind back to the okra scene. *Ffffzzzzhhhh!* Okay, here we are:

. . . I raised my own fork to my mouth. *(SMELLY OKRA, MUSHY OKRA, CRUSTY OKRA, GAG!)* I took a bite and chewed and swallowed and—hark! What heaven is in mine mouth? Can this be the slimy okra? The okra of seedy and wet? It was, and it was damn good! I had several more helpings of Catherine's okra that night. The very next day I secured my own stash of okra, I cooked it according to Catherine's directions, and we ate it every night for a month. I used to look forward to the summers when the farmers' markets are flush with silk-tressed ears of corn, but okra is the new corn. It doesn't even need to be logrolled in butter, pepper, and salt; all it takes is a bit of olive oil and salt, and it's completely and utterly delicious.

There was no question of not eating the okra, in case you were wondering. My inflexible politeness, while absent during my growing-up years, is now so intractable that it does not allow me to politely refuse to eat food at other people's houses. Because then they'd *know*. And at this stage in my life, I am way more afraid of drawing attention to my pickiness and eliciting mental eye rolls than I am of the food itself. I am also just as fearful of putting my hosts out with my pickiness. I certainly don't want them trying to find something else for me to eat just because of my issues.

My seduction to the Okra Side is just one example of how my inbred manners forced me to eat foods out of politeness—foods that required me to take deep breaths, perform a six-point gag reflex check, and keep my hand on a glass of water for an emergency wash-down—only to discover a deep and abiding love for said foods.

That's what my mannerly upbringing did for me, and I'm grateful to my parents for that. But not everyone is so lucky. There are some picky eaters who can't even contemplate the idea of having the food in their mouth, much less chewing and swallowing, without tensing up or retching. I can relate to all of that, so what do you do when faced with the dreaded dinner party invitation? What's the picky eating etiquette?

Under the heading, "Problems at the Dinner Table," *The*

Amy Vanderbilt Complete Book of Etiquette offers this advice: "If you find there is something in your mouth you cannot eat, like a piece of gristle, do not spit it into your napkin. Instead, put your fork up to your mouth and remove the inedible object; replace it on your plate where you can bury it under some food so it is not visible." That's not exactly something you can do with an entire serving of "something you cannot eat," and since Amy also notes elsewhere that "Many single women feel quite secure about entertaining on their own. However, asking a man friend to act as cohost for the evening can be helpful and reassuring," I'm thinking she might not be the one to turn to for advice in the new millennium.

For a picky perspective beyond my own Grin and Try Not to Gag on It approach, I turn to my friend Keith, who might have the distinction of being the pickiest person I know and who famously won't eat anything green except green M&M's. Keith tells me that most people know him well enough to know how picky he is. Those friends, he says, are often kind enough to ask what they should prepare. However, in other situations—like a party—where it's not feasible to plan around everyone's diets and preferences, Keith simply doesn't eat. He explains, "I'll either politely refuse or simply pretend to be eating by spreading a bunch of food around my plate. I definitely try not to impose on the hosts." If he's worried that there won't be enough for him to eat, Keith will eat a big snack ahead of time or eat something after. While Keith admits that there are times he wishes he could be less picky "in order to be able to eat more socially," he seems pretty comfortable with his pickiness and not at all ashamed of something that wasn't his biological choice. Dr. Zucker would be proud of him.

In addition to picky eaters accepting who they are and not

being ashamed of it, I'd also like to see more hosts and hostesses be sympathetic enough to ask their guests ahead of time if there are any foods they don't eat, which is how I phrase it. I know exactly how it feels to sit through a meal with a stomach twisted into miserable little dread knots. The easily annoyed might not like this idea, as they huff over how impossible it is to cater to everyone's dislikes. My only response is that I've never had a problem planning a meal around what people don't eat. My formerly picky friend Sam, who makes a point of serving her dinners family style, which allows her guests to choose how much of each dish they want for themselves, actually sees planning a restricted meal as a creative challenge.

But reality dictates that not every host is going to ask. Some—maybe most—hosts are going to cook the food and expect you to eat it. And not every picky eater is going to be as comfortable as Keith politely refusing food. I'm not going to show you how to eat—that'll be attempted in another chapter—but how to survive.

The Picky Eater's Guide to Surviving a Dinner Party

Most—if not all—of these methods have been rigorously tested by yours truly. Admittedly, the majority of them were implemented when I was a kid, but consider this: It was harder for me to get away with these things as a kid because my beleaguered parents maintained constant vigilance at/under the dinner table and in the kitchen. And bathrooms. And windows.

1. **Baked Potato Skins:** Just like those hide-a-key rocks from Brookstone, baked potato skins allow you to hide unwanted food practically in plain sight. My older sister and I hit upon the Potato Skin Escape Hatch once my parents gave up on insisting that we eat our (allegedly) vitamin-packed skins. Once you have secretly filled the empty baked potato skin with unwanted food, the key is to strategically crush the skin with the back of a spoon (we used the heel of our hands, but that's harder to pull off when you're an adult) in order to give the skin the appearance of being empty. And unless you have a host who—like my freak husband—decides to eat your "empty" potato skin off your plate, you're home free.

   Picky Pro Tip: *To make sure baked potatoes are on the menu that night, seed advance conversations with your host about how much you love baked potatoes. If your host considers herself a consummate cook, try bemoaning the fact that no one really knows how to make a proper baked potato and that you are on a quest to find the perfect one. Take it from a cook who knows, your host will try to deliver a perfect baked potato unto you.*

2. **Paper Napkins:** Sure, this is a crude tactic, but probably one of the oldest and goodliest. It worked for many years in my house and is as simple as: napkin in lap, food in lap, food in napkin. Ball the napkin up into your fist and toss at your earliest convenience. It's best to stash in yours or your wife's purse (plastic baggies come in handy here, too) and deal with outside of

your host's home, but the kitchen trash is acceptable, too.

Picky Pro Tip: *Invest in cargo pants. The more pockets, the better.*

Drawback: *Fancy friends who only use cloth napkins.*

3. **Escherize Your Plate:** This is more than just pushing your food around your plate. This takes it to another level. An optical illusion level. What you need to do is find the arrangement that makes the same amount of food *look* like there's less on the plate. And it needs to look natural. Lining your plate with a circumference of peas will make it look like you have fewer peas, but it will also make you look like a freak, which is exactly what we're trying to avoid. (Looking over my shoulder at my laptop screen as I write this, Mark informs me, "The Banach-Tarski Theorem uses actual mathematics to prove that there is a way to cut an object into a finite number of pieces and rearrange it into something half the size." He adds, "I mean, it's true that no one's ever *actually* done it, but the point is that it's been proven that it can be done." Hope springs eternal.)

Picky Pro Tip: *Practice at home, and when you get arrangements that could work in a variety of situations, take photos of them with your cell phone of choice, and then refer to those pictures at the dinner party. You won't look any ruder than the people checking email, Twittering their Four Squares, and sending texts.*

4. **Bookshelves:** Maybe they have books in the kitchen, maybe they have them in the living room, but wherever they are, find them and use them to your advantage by sticking food behind the volumes of David Foster Wallace, Colette, and Stephenie Meyer. If noticed, your literary loitering will just make you look so high-minded that mere food—such a crass mortal addiction!—can't pull you away from your intellectual pursuits. My sister proudly pioneered this tactic in our house, and my mother is still finding fossilized hamburgers to this day.

Picky Pro Tip: *Know ahead of time which books they've already read and are therefore least likely to pull out anytime soon.*

Drawback: *Doesn't work in houses of the illiterate.*

5. **Get Pregnant (Sorry, Guys):** Pregnant women get a pass on just about everything, especially food. When you are "great with child," food aversions are very real and documented events. The scientists tell me that food aversion during pregnancy probably occurs because the baby is telling the mother what it wants (and who can argue with a Cheetos-craving fetus? I couldn't) and doesn't want (in my case: fresh vegetables, fish, and anything healthy).

6. **Yoga:** As you know, Dr. Zucker is big on relaxing the body before sitting down for a meal to combat food anxiety, so don't be afraid to unfurl a sticky mat in the

middle of the kitchen and do a few Down Dogs or Sun Salutations to bring yourself to a calm center. Everyone will admire your dedication to your spiritual and physical well-being and wish they were so disciplined.

> **Picky Pro Tip:** *To further the effect and reduce even more anxiety, throw some Oms into table conversation. For example, "Ooohhhmmm going to need a wine refill," "Ooohhhmmmazing weather we're having, don't you think?" and "You know, ooohhhmmmbilical cords are crazy things—they're like a straw in the uterus!"*

7. **Offer to Clean the Kitchen.** Look what a great guest you are! You are giving your fatigued host a break from the kitchen where they've been slaving away all day and clearing everyone's plates, including yours! The best way to effect this maneuver is to be mindful of when dinner is drawing to a close. Immediately, drop your napkin over your plate, all casual-like, and pick up your plate before anyone can really get a good look at what's left. (This is where cloth napkins work best.) Announce that you are volunteering to clean up and suggest that everyone stay in their seats and enjoy the surprise dessert you brought over. (Note: Bring a surprise dessert.) If another guest tries to hone in on your generosity, divert them by suggesting they serve your surprise dessert, leaving you in peace to deal with the food.

> **Drawback:** *You will probably get invited back.*

8. **Urns.** This is not for the fainthearted. But come on, big urn just sitting there mostly empty? And seriously, who is going to check it? By the way, if you do try this and get caught, drop some ancient Egyptian burial knowledge on your hosts and demand to know why their dearly departed doesn't deserve to have food in the afterlife like King Tut. Announce you were treating the deceased like royalty, and then end by telling them they're lucky you didn't stuff the cat in there, too.

Drawback: You probably won't get invited back.

Author's Note: Admittedly, this is not one I have personally tried, but only because my mother won't tell us where she hid my grandparents. However, I did get the idea from an episode of Mad About You, *and Paul Reiser is very trustworthy.*

And then send your host a huge bouquet of flowers the next day to thank them for such a wonderful meal. After all, they will find your new additions to their library one day.

Much easier than the dinner party for the picky eater is dining out at a restaurant. At least here, picky eaters have a modicum of control over what they eat, and unless you're like me, you don't have to worry about offending the people who made the food. However, restaurants can still be scary for picky eaters. Maybe educating both camps can help smooth the way for all, but first some introductions are in order.

Picky Eater, Meet Chef

Chefs are culinary architects. When they create a dish, every component of that dish is there for a reason.

Under consideration for the chef are visual presentation, complementary flavors, texture, and balance. Bearing that in mind, it's understandable that chefs aren't always so thrilled when diners want to muck around with their creations, especially when they think any substitutions or subtractions might compromise the final outcome of the dish and, as a result, also compromise your enjoyment of it. Using the simple example of tomatoes, most chefs would agree that all tomatoes—no matter how ripe, local, or heirloomed they may be—taste better with salt. I believe it might have been Julia Child who said, "Salt makes tomatoes taste like tomatoes." Therefore, without the simple inclusion of salt, tomatoes can taste bland, dull, uninteresting.

You can enlarge the example if you think about a slightly more complex example, like tomato sauce, which, at its most basic, calls for olive oil, onion, carrots, oregano, tomato paste, tomatoes, garlic, basil, salt, and pepper. Each component contributes something to the overall dish. Each component builds flavor. Remove one of them and you have a different dish, a different flavor. Chefs know how flavors and ingredients react to one another. Some play nice, some dominate the other ingredients, some fall in love, and some beat each other up so badly that they can't be in the same dish together. It is understandable that chefs get miffed when someone messes with their masterpiece. After all, it is their job to know what will be most delicious to most people.

Chef, Meet Picky Eater

However, chefs also need to remember that they are in the business of service and their ultimate goal should be to make their diners happy. Egos get involved when chefs think they know more than the customer about what will most please them. On the whole, I'd say chefs are correct, and I personally put my trust in them. But when it comes to picky eating, chefs need to try to comprehend how one particular inclusion of an offensive (to the picky eater) ingredient can take over and ruin the entire dish for them. The chef may have created the dish with balance in mind, but for a picky eater, there is no balance in a dish if the only thing the picky diner can taste is that one despised ingredient.

Some of my friends are very set against reading restaurant menus in advance of an upcoming meal, because it ruins the surprise for them. I'll give you 10 to 1 odds that those are the people who aren't and never have been picky eaters, because when it comes to food, picky eaters don't like surprises. Picky eaters especially don't like a menu item with the word "surprise" in it, which is usually code for something that is stuffed with an amorphous mass of indiscernible composition and suspicious origin. I suppose we should count ourselves lucky that having live birds fly out of huge pies hasn't been fashionable for about five hundred years. Surprises, unexpected encounters with ingredients not listed on the menu, or running into raisins where none were thought to exist . . . these don't excite us; they freak us out. Picky eaters live a more straightforward existence, and while it might not be full of *Indiana Jones* culinary adventures where bugs or monkey brains are consumed, we're pretty okay with that. However, even with the existence of online menus to prepare the picky eater for what lies ahead, dining out can still be fraught with pitfalls and mantraps.

Amy Watts, a recovering picky eater, tells me about a nightmarish preinterview dinner she had with a future boss. They went to a local restaurant, where Amy was terrified there would be nothing she could order that would result in her being able to eat every last scrap on her plate. Eating every last smear, scrap, or garnish on her plate was very important to Amy because while she had usually done the *When Harry Met Sally* dance of, "I want this but leave this off and put this on the side," she didn't want her future boss to look at her and think, "Picky eater!" "Because of the social stigma," Amy explains. Although she admits she didn't eat her asparagus, she at least found something she could order without modifying it. However, when they went to a Southwestern-Asian fusion restaurant the next day, Amy thought, "Great! Things that scare the crap out of me all on one menu!" and sought refuge in a grilled cheese sandwich. "Because," Amy concludes, "grilled cheese is the safest thing a picky eater can order."

Like Amy, I didn't like doing the *When Harry Met Sally* dance at restaurants either, and in fact, I never did it. But my worries were less about what was going through my dining companions' minds and more fixated on what the waiter or kitchen staff thought of me. I didn't want to be high maintenance or a burden. I didn't want to put anyone out to cater to my "special needs." In fact, I was so worried about offending the kitchen with any uneaten food on my plate that if I didn't want to eat my side vegetables, I'd quickly sneak them onto Mark's plate and urge him to eat them while no one was looking. I had this idea—somewhat borne out of self-conscious paranoia but also supported by angry chef and waiter blogs—that restaurant folks were pretty disdainful of customers in general and picky eaters in particular. When I went to a restaurant, I never sent things back and I never asked for substitutions or made special requests. I kept my head down, pawned off broccoli on Mark, and hoped that nothing I did would lead me to question whether the spittle on my dessert really was a product of molecular gastronomy or a sign of the restaurant staff's scorn.

Do restaurant workers really hate picky eaters so much they'd spit in their food? Is there a way picky eaters should behave in a restaurant while still being able to enjoy their meals? I decide to bust into the steamy restaurants of San Francisco and find out the truth once and for all pickykind. And while I'm at it, I might as well educate the restaurants about picky eaters. You know, tell them about genetics and psychology and sword-swallowing so they might understand where their picky customers are coming from. I will be a picky eating evangelist, spreading the food word straight from the church of Our Lady of Perpetual Gagging! I'll probably need a bell.

Among my experts of choice are Brett and Elan Emerson, co-owners of Contigo, a Spanish and Catalan restaurant in San Francisco's sun-steeped Noe Valley neighborhood, and Michael Procopio, a mustachioed waiter with twenty years of feeding the public under his apron.

Brett, the head chef and owner of a restaurant that features pig trotters, tripe, oxtail, anchovies, and sardines, is himself a former picky eater and perhaps it's because of that perspective that he actually shies away from the term "picky." "'Picky' has negative connotations. People have preferences. I don't really have a problem with people having different preferences," Brett explains. Some of his customers will order the pig trotters and sardines, but others order a salad and *albóndigas* (Spanish meatballs). "And that's what Contigo is to them. They don't even notice the other things, or if they do, they never order them, but I don't judge them either way. As long as they come in and eat something."

Similarly, Michael also exorcises my visions of an impatient server tapping his pen irritably against his pad as he manages to both roll his eyes and check his watch in abject annoyance with my halting explanation of how raisins, bananas, oatmeal, cream of wheat, grits, polenta, the skin of tomatoes, caviar, offal, innards, feet, flan, tofu, red peppers, yellow peppers, cooked green peppers, cooked green beans, some fish, figs, dates, most melon, stews, braises, gelatinous desserts, rabbit, veal, dill, black licorice, tarragon, lemongrass, coleslaw, mozzarella cheese, mayonnaise, rice pudding, some leafy greens, cooked cherries, fruit-flavored chocolate, peas and carrots in fried rice, tapioca, cream sauces, and anything wrapped in grape leaves or seaweed must never come near me.

"It's not a big deal for me," Michael tells me over lunch. When I tell him that I've heard of instances where waiters and waitresses won't even check with the kitchen before flatly denying a diner's request, his response was convincing. "They're just lazy," he pronounces decidedly, adding, "It's my job to give people what they need."

"But how should a picky eater behave?" I ask. "To, you know, not piss anyone off?"

1. Ask and maybe ye shall not receive

As the restaurant's manager, Elan is in charge of every aspect of Contigo's service. This includes the folks who are on the finicky frontlines, the waitstaff. For her part, Elan simply wants customers to be honest and clear. "As restaurateurs, we need people to communicate what they like and don't like, and then we can tell them whether or not we can accommodate them."

Elan trains Contigo's waitstaff to be familiar with all the dishes so that if a diner has mentioned their dislikes, the staff can guide them away from something and perhaps toward another choice. "That's my dream: that the servers can help guide, and that they take care of the diner throughout the entire dinner, so when they are dropping the food, they are saying, 'No egg in this one,' or whatever, to the particular diner."

Contigo's kitchen actually changed the way they prepared a dish because of how frequently customers asked for certain subtractions. Originally, the dish—sautéed greens with pine nuts and raisins—called for combining the toasted pine nuts and soaked raisins ahead of time and en masse. This meant that if the customer wanted the greens without the raisins or without the pine nuts, it couldn't be done. However, because of how frequently Brett and Elan got requests for "no nuts" or "without the raisins," the pine nuts and raisins are added separately to the greens after the order is placed. In this situation, it ended up being easier to adapt their prep in order to better accommodate their guests. How wonderful that a restaurant would go to such lengths to please their customers. I mean, it's like they *care* or something!

Elan is shocked when I tell her I would simply avoid a dish with raisins in it. "You wouldn't just say something?" she says, her eyes round with disbelief. Well, I will *now*.

Michael has a similar response. He also tells me he wants picky eaters to behave honestly. "As long as they're clear about it, and we both know what is going to happen, I'm completely fine about it," he adds.

2. Stick to the menu

As noted earlier, the proliferation of online menus makes being a picky eater in this digital age just a little bit easier; do some research and know what you're getting into before you get to the restaurant.

At Contigo, Brett is so conscious of his customers' preferences that he goes out of his way to make sure the menu lists the ingredients of each dish whenever possible. Brett admits that it's not always possible to list every single ingredient, so for the more complex dishes he tries at the very least to hit the allergens or the "really quirky things," such as raisins or tomatoes.

While some restaurants might be able to whip you up something that isn't on their menu, most of them don't have the time or necessary ingredients to cater to off-menu requests. So don't go ordering a cheeseburger at a Vietnamese restaurant, then get huffy when they can't comply.

And on that huffy note . . .

3. Be polite: you can catch more flies with maple syrup[1]

Some chefs have told me their impressions of picky eaters are diners who are demanding, entitled, and imperious about their preferences. The kind of customers who act as though their

---

1. I don't like honey.

dislikes simply serve to show how elite and rarified a palate they have. Now, I personally haven't run into any of those types of picky eaters in my life or research, but that doesn't mean they don't exist. So here's a tip: Don't be rude about your dislikes or preferences. Don't be rude, period. Don't make faces, stick out your tongue, grab your throat and gag—none of that.[2]

I wouldn't have thought this was something that anyone above the age of eight needed to be told, but Michael has actually gotten the grossed-out reaction from diners when he describes a dish. "And they haven't even seen it!" he says incredulously. Even if your insides quake at the idea of goat stew, do what you can to keep it all inside. Not doing so makes the rest of us look bad and gives weight to the misconception that adult picky eaters are childish, immature, and need to grow up.

4. Be aware of your surroundings

If the restaurant is packed or it's a weekend night, it might be harder for the cooks to accommodate certain special requests. It's not that they don't want to, Elan explains, but part of her job does involve protecting the kitchen, and she can't grind the kitchen to a halt on a busy night because of a special request.

5. Know how the sausage is made

Restaurants do a lot of advance preparation to make sure food gets out to their customers as quickly as possible, so there

---

2. And remember what Dr. Zucker said about making gross-out faces: It clenches your stomach and makes it unreceptive to food.

might be some recipes that simply cannot be changed. For instance, items such as meatballs or crab cakes are made ahead of time, so if they happen to contain something you're averse to—onions, peppers, dill, etc.—the kitchen can't modify that for you. It's better to move on to something else. Other things that might be made in bulk are risotto, soups, stews, vinaigrettes for salads, and sauces.

Try to be as flexible as you can, and don't get your heart set on one dish so that you are left panicking and sweating about what to order if it can't be modified. Most important, when in doubt, talk it through with your server.

6. Avoid a case of mistaken identity

The restaurateur's request not to falsely represent your food preferences is a valid one, but it requires a little more of the picky eating perspective than the others. There are picky eaters who hide behind their own definition of allergies and vegetarianism, which prompts the request from Elan, "Don't come in and say you're vegetarian, but eat chicken," or that you have ambiguous and undiagnosed food "allergies."[3] Both of these excuses have the side effect of obfuscating the truth and confusing the restaurant staff, who are there to guide you through your meal. "I can't help you if you mislabel your preference," Elan explains.

---

3. I'm not talking about actual food allergies, like celiac disease and nut allergies.

"Allergies"

Let's face it, most picky eaters (including, dear reader, myself) who cry allergy do so because it's far more socially acceptable to claim a medical condition than to bleat, "I don't like peppers." Like my friend Chi-An, who told me her tomato aversion "provoked a physical reaction, at least as strong as [her] actual medical allergies," I believed that bell peppers made me physically ill with nauseous migraines. (It could have been a bell pepper intolerance, but this was fifteen years ago, when the distinction between food allergies and food *intolerances* wasn't causing all-caps foodie screaming fights on Twitter.) And it's possible that I willed that reaction in myself because of just how much I hated the lousy things, but the fact of the matter is, I retreated behind the protective barrier of an "allergy" because it was easy. It was an excuse that no one in polite society would question.

Michael, however, informs me how wrong I was. As a waiter, he takes food allergies very seriously, and is well aware of customers who claim to have an allergy when it's actually just a dislike. "And I play along, because what am I going to do? Call them out in front of their friends? My tip depends on it!" Apparently, those of us with food "allergies" aren't fooling anyone.

Furthermore, with all the medically defined allergies and intolerances out there today—nuts, gluten, lactose, shellfish, etc.—the genuinely allergic would probably appreciate it if the picky eaters would stop using their excuse, which has the unfortunate side effect of diluting their own legitimate claims. Instead of claiming a nonexistent "allergy," say you have an intolerance, aversion, or bad reaction to the food in question. At the very least, "intolerance" or "bad reaction" conjures up visions of mad dashes to the bathroom, which will get the subject dropped quite quickly.

"Vegetarians"

I've come across a lot of people who are vegetarians for reasons other than the PETA-inspired, ethical standpoint. There are those who can't digest meat of any kind. Others have bad reactions to beef and therefore find it easier to cut out all meat than have to ask, "But what kind of stock is it cooked in?" or "Do you use beef fat for frying these vegetables?" Then there's my friend Lora, who, if she had a choice, would eat meat. "I actually like meat," she confesses, "I just can't."

Lora tells people she's vegetarian for simplicity's sake, but she actually defines herself as a "weirdly picky eater." Claiming vegetarianism is much easier than getting into all the gory details, because Lora's problem is that she can't stop herself from seeing the animal in its original, alive, non-marinated form. As a kid who briefly lived on a farm, Lora had the misfortune to see decapitated chickens run around spewing blood, she played with a bunny that later ended up on her plate, and she heard lobsters scream from a pot as they got the life boiled out of them.[4] If Lora had lived on that farm for more than three months, she might have gotten to the point where she saw dead animals as food and not just dead animals. Instead: "I didn't get to work through it. I got to see the bloody, running chickens. And they run—do you, have

---

4. Actually, lobsters don't scream. According to Dr. Robert Bayer, a professor of animal and veterinary sciences and the executive director of the Lobster Institute at the University of Maine, "Lobsters have no means of vocalization." Well, then, what was it that Lora heard? "Sometimes air is trapped in the stomach and may come out during cooking, making a sound." Kind of sounds like they're burping more than anything else. But try telling that to a freaked-out second grader and see how far you get.

you ever? They *move*," Lora says, dropping her voice to a hor-rified whisper.

So far, this does sound like a lot of other vegetarians who have ethical reasons why they won't eat animals. However, Lora's brand of picky eating becomes even more complicated because of a self-defensive loophole that allows her to eat some meaty things. "I kind of have this ridiculous rule that if it's ugly, and it would hurt me, then I can eat it." (Interest-ingly, this is the opposite of other picky eaters who would refuse to eat something *because* it's so ugly it actually grosses them out.[5]) Salmon, Lora tells me, falls into this category because it has teeth and is ugly. However, sharks are a no-go because she finds them "strangely beautiful."

Although I won't eat rabbit because they remind me too much of my cats, Lora's story is a new one to me, but she's not alone in her "vegetarianism." In fact, when she has been pressed to explain the reasons behind her vegetarianism, she has found many kindred spirits who can't eat meat for the exact same reasons and have a hard time explaining it to people without having PETA accusations flung at them.

Unless you really are a full-on vegetarian, I'd suggest drop-ping the word "vegetarian" completely. Otherwise, it brings up complicating questions relating to stock or broth choice, foods touching or being cooked on the same surface as meat, etc. Simply say, "The only meat I eat is chicken."

(However, for those like Lora who are up to telling their

---

5. In an effort to create drama, an episode of the competitive cooking show *Top Chef* intentionally grossed out kids by showing them a dead monkfish before serving it to them.

whole story, I say give it to them with both barrels. Ask: "Do you have any ugly, dangerous meat on your menu tonight? Because that's the only kind of meat I can eat."

Clear, honest communication, just like Elan requested.)

Sitting there in Contigo's empty dining room as the staff prepared for dinner, I finally ask the question that's been troubling me from the beginning of the interview: "Have you ever been tempted to spit into a diner's food?" Shocked by my question, Brett busts out laughing, shaking his head and waving his hands in denial, and Elan gasps, "No! Oh, *no!*"

Unfortunately, while Brett and Elan Emerson and Michael Procopio are all kind, understanding restaurant people who put their customers' desires first, there are other chefs out there who aren't as sympathetic. One local and infamously opinionated chef initially agreed to meet with me to discuss picky eaters and restaurant manners but then changed his mind within hours, telling me the subject was a sore one for him and he was going to have to pass. I can only guess what the content of that interview would have been like, but I don't think it would have been filled with the milk of human kindness.

However, picky eaters shouldn't let that sort of chef scare them from eating out. Stand picky, stand proud.

(And eat at Contigo.)

CHAPTER 8

Love and the Picky Eater

Crystalline tears streaked down her alabaster cheeks. Her smooth and perfectly shaven armpits were moistening with the delicate sweat of a stuck pig and would soon soak the grass green T-shirt she had dressed herself in just that morning. "Mercy me!" she choked out, carefully tapping the corners of her mouth with a hand-stitched velvet napkin. "That's hot!" He turned his magnificent visage in her direction and looked at her with eyes that bored into her very soul. "Is it . . . too hot?" he asked with great concern in those eyes that she suddenly and hungrily realized were as brown and sweet as the richest hot chocolate in France. Her breast heaved as she gulped down ice-cold water from a crystal goblet. The water streamed out of the sides of her pouty red lips and made her T-shirt stick to her in big wet patches. "Oh, no, it's just great!" she said as her piquantly tipped nose streamed large snot globules that were as glistening and white as the purest of pearls the deepest ocean oyster had to offer. That was the first lie she told to her future husband.

That night, she sat and gazed at the stone-hewn walls of his

Trinity College room and lifted each forkful of pepper-riddled
pasta to her ruby red lips, which were swollen in reaction to the
red sauce he had personally doctored with large pinches from a
vial inscribed with a label that read "Lucianovic's Powdered Fire."
As she thirstily drank in chiseled cheeks and thick dark hair that
her slender fingers ached to twine, she knew that she could never
tell him the truth about herself. He could never know the deep,
dark secret she kept buried in the pit of her stomach. After all,
she had kept mum on the subject for years. This tall, dashing
mathematician could never know that she was a picky eater.

Crushes, infatuations, and love make us do the damnedest
things. I once baked dirt into brownies (on purpose) as part
of a "spell" I was "casting" on an eighth-grade crush. (It didn't
work.) And then there were the six years I sent my friend's
older brother anonymous, handmade Valentines. (It's not
stalking if paper doilies are involved.) However, the craziest
thing I ever did for love was eat.

But first I was going to lie through my teeth about it.

Picky eaters know that being picky is an extremely unattractive personality trait, as sure to purge the romance out
of any relationship as a massive chin zit or a past involvement
with the KKK. To many, being unable to eat certain foods,
for whatever reason, makes someone unlovable. "Immature!"
"Narrow-minded!" "Hopelessly unsophisticated!" Those are
just a sampling of the descriptors picky eaters can see popping
open above a date's head like cartoon word bubbles once the
date is let in on the picky secret. And thanks to *When Harry
Met Sally*, picky eaters can also add "high maintenance" to
the list.

Examples of picky eating as an unattractive trait abound in pop culture and literature, but here are a few standouts:

SEALed with a Kiss: Romance Novel

It was surprising to learn that a picky eater was featured in a romance novel about Navy SEALs, so of course that meant it needed to be fully researched.[1] In this book, the hero, a Navy SEAL, notes how persnickety the heroine is about food. Among other examples, he observes her asking lots of questions about prepared food items in a grocery store, turning one after another down, and this "high-maintenance" quality manages to squelch his ardor, albeit temporarily. When he later learns that she's not actually picky or watching her weight, and instead has celiac disease, it's all good. Because that's a medical complaint, and she implies she might die if she's not careful. Still, the takeaway message is that picky eating is not a desirable trait if you hope to snag a SEAL and have sex in a swing.

Picky-Picky: Cat

"Picky-Picky," a sobriquet that all but damned the poor thing to an unloved existence, is Ramona Quimby's grumpy old cat in the Beverly Cleary books. After Picky-Picky stays true to

---

1. The cover alone is worth a look—dog tags glinting off an extremely muscular, highly polished SEAL chest.

his name by turning his whiskered nose up at cheaper brands of cat food, he grows so ravenous that he snacks on and ruins the family's carefully carved jack-o'-lantern. Picky-Picky is portrayed more as a nuisance than as a beloved member of the family. Only Beezus seems to actually give a crap about that cat, and given that she is a grumpy older sister, her affection is not exactly a ringing endorsement for feline lovability.

When Harry Met Sally: Movie

Finally, there's *When Harry Met Sally.* Sure, Harry eventually marries Sally, touts her pickiness as a positive thing when he's setting her up with Bruno Kirby—"She orders [food] in a way that even the chef didn't know how good it could be!"—and even seems to come around to her way of thinking, but that's only *after* twelve years of playing Pictionary, faking deli orgasms, and singing "Surrey with the Fringe on Top" in front of Ira. The first time Harry meets Sally, her personality tic of "wanting it the way [she] wants it" plays as something unattractive or annoying.

Sally, in all her "on the side" glory, is an Honest Picky Eater, because there are two types of picky eaters on the dating scene: the Lying Picky Eater and the Honest Picky Eater. Fully aware that their admirable honesty might result in heartbreak, the Honest Picky Eater is up front about the foods she doesn't like or how she wants her food prepared. The Lying Picky Eater, on the other hand, will do anything to avoid revealing her secret identity, including going so far as to actually *eat* the hated foods.

The Honest Picky Eater has a strong sense of self. She

might not even be ashamed of being picky. It's who she is, she can't help it, and if you can't take her—food aversions and all—well, you can just ask for the check and leave. (I doff my hat to them. Stand picky, stand proud.) The Lying Picky Eater, on the other hand, is way more afraid of what people will think of him than he is of eating the food. (The Lying Picky Eater probably has better control over his gag reflex, too.)

I was a Lying Picky Eater. I was going keep my picky eating under wraps for as long as possible. Forever, if necessary. I would bury the awful truth as deeply as I buried my despised falafel dinner at canoe camp. Amy Watts was a Lying Picky Eater, too. Such was her embarrassment over her pickiness that when a guy she had a crush on presented her with a horrifying bowl of freshly picked strawberries, she ate them.

Lying Picky Eaters will eat foods they hate or fear in the same way other people might suck in their stomachs or bleach their teeth. The plan is to hide the flaw until that special someone loves them too much to care that they can't stand it when their fish touches their sweet potatoes, which they wouldn't even have on their plates in the first place because they hate things that swim in the ocean or are orange. Believe me, if picky eaters had our own Cyrano de Bergerac we could smuggle in under our coats to eat all our food for us on dates, we'd do it. (Instead of a big nose, he'd have a big mouth, which is actually sort of creepy when you think about it.)

Picky eaters are eternally put on the dating defensive. I've heard people say, "I wouldn't date a picky eater," but I've never heard anyone say, "I would never date a foodie." Why? Because picky eaters are made to feel that their way is the wrong way, and that indiscriminately eating everything from fish that siphon the ocean of all its crap to the organs that are put in animals specifically to get rid of all their crap is the right way. On behalf of picky eaters everywhere, I'm going to go on the picky offensive for once. I'm going to strike a blow for all pickykind and say that if you won't date a picky eater, you are anti-Semitic.

That's right, I'm about to go biblical on your ass.

After Moses led the Israelites out of Egypt and away from Pharaoh's grasp, they had only a few weeks' enjoyment of their wandering freedom before the former slaves got a bit peckish and whiny. God heard them and sent sustenance in the form of manna. The Bible variously describes manna as tasting like oil, cakes cooked in oil, or wafers dipped in honey.[2] However, the picture tacked up on the wall of my Sunday school classroom showed Moses and his people foraging what looked to me like cotton candy. (That is, Moses' people foraged. In every piece of art I've seen, it looks like Moses did a whole lot of directing and not much actual picking of stuff off the ground.)

I initially thought it would be pretty exciting to discover that it had rained carnival food overnight—until I learned that the fleeing Israelites had to eat the manna for forty years. Forty days would have been bad enough (and God knows there are plenty of those increments in the Bible), but forty years? Not only that, but if any of the Israelites were greedy and took more manna than they or their family would consume in a day (perhaps hoping to store up a bit in lean times),

---

2. Wording depends on your version. I prefer the King James; it's verbose and requires a dictionary, but it's also very lyrical and pretty, which is especially nice when reading about death and destruction.

they'd find that their celestial leftovers had rotted and become infested with worms overnight. It was their punishment for not trusting the chef, i.e., God, to provide them with enough food each day. In a sense, God with His manna was the exact opposite of Joan Crawford in *Mommie Dearest* pulling out the same plate of uneaten food and forcing it on Christina for breakfast, lunch, and dinner. Then again, Joan Crawford didn't drop a plague on her kids. (But only because she didn't think of it. Probably.)

Apparently, forty years of manna was a bit much for the Israelites, too, because after one Mannaloaf Night too many, a bunch of them—a group that the Oxford Annotated Bible calls "rabble"—whined to Moses about wanting "flesh" and how they missed all the fish, cucumbers, garlic, leeks, and onions they had in Egypt. You know, in the good old days when they were slaves. Moses took their complaints and his own (because you know he was just as tired as they were of Zipporah's creative uses for manna, especially her Manna Surprise, which was just "Surprise, more manna!") to God, who got royally pissed off by their ungrateful pickiness. God darkly promised that He would provide them with flesh to eat, quite a bit of flesh, actually. He promised they would eat flesh for a month "until it come out at your nostrils, and it be loathsome unto you." That's gross enough, but then when God sent them the promised nostril-filling flesh, He doled out additional punishment in the form of a plague and killed a bunch of Israelites. All for being Honest Picky Eaters. And thus, we could say that picky eaters have long suffered for their singular palate—they never even got to the Promised Land.

Ergo, not dating a picky eater = anti-Semitic.

"You don't remember, do you?" Mark asks me after I triumphantly read my latest picky conspiracy theory to him.

"What?" I ask.

"The time you asked if I was a 'food snob.'"

"I did not."

"You did! You totally did! We were just talking about our dinner—we were at an Indian restaurant—and you stopped me and demanded, 'Wait, are you a food snob?! You are! *You're a food snob!*' And inside, I was thinking, 'Duh, *of course!*' but I didn't want to say that out loud to you, because I was definitely worried that this was along the lines of someone asking me, 'Are you a Trekkie?' and it would be the last I saw of you."

"Wait, so you were worried about what I thought of your eating habits?"

"I started sweating, I was on the defensive."

Damn, let she who is without sin cast the first stonefruit.

"If you're in the dating process, and food is a deal breaker, you're probably not going in the right direction to start with," Jim McKinney tells me over the phone. "Mmm-hmm!" Anne agrees forcefully from another extension. Jim and Anne McKinney are old friends of my mother and father-in-law and have been married for forty-seven years. I sought their advice and perspective as an example of a mixed-food couple from another generation.

Anne loves eating, cooking, and experimenting with food. Jim, on the other hand, doesn't call himself a picky eater, but he definitely is selective compared to his wife. "There are certain things I won't eat," Jim explains, outing himself as an Honest Picky Eater, "and I think Anne accepts that, and as long as it's not the majority of the food on planet Earth, then I think we're in good shape." Over the years, Anne has finessed

Jim to the point where the only things he won't eat are mushrooms, olives, peppers, and seafood. And when Anne makes something new, Jim does try it. "She'll run a campaign on a food item, like quinoa," Jim explains. "She'll point out an article—in the back of her mind she knows she's going to make this—she'll tell me it will make my hair curly, and it's going to be good for me. So, she'll lay the groundwork and voilà! It will show up." In the most basic way, Jim and Anne weren't the perfect food match, but even so they never had a "you're going to have to change the way you eat" conversation. "It's silly to get into an argument about food. It just is," Jim concludes.

Except that we *do* get into arguments about food. In fact, because we have more options and choices than we ever did before, we might argue even more about food today than we ever did before. Whatever your culinary camp—organic, locavore, vegan, omnivore, picky—you can bet people have passionately argued for and against it. They've delivered papers on the subject, written books, and probably protested in its name. Everyone is convinced that their way is the "right" way, and that the poor benighted individuals who dare to have an opposing opinion are flat-out wrong.

Maybe some people can let the food differences go, spread their hands wide, and say, "It's all good. We can still get along even though we're different—the world is a rainbow, man!" But others can't, and it does end up affecting their relationships.

". . . and then he said his favorite restaurant was Citizen Cake, so you know that's going nowhere," my friend Jen said, matter-of-factly summing up a date to me as we hacked our way through the damp, green trails of Lands End one foggy

San Francisco afternoon. I nodded sympathetically, knowing exactly what she meant. Jen's Citizen Cake statement is not one of snobbery; it's about food compatibility. There are a lot of potential incompatible food couples out there: koshers and non-koshers, vegans and carnivores, foodies and pickies. Jen is a foodie—though all foodies hate that term, we have yet to come up with an acceptable replacement that sticks[3]—and finding someone with whom she is compatible, food-wise, is important to her.

It is difficult to understand why food compatibility can be more polarizing in relationships than, say, having a similar taste in books. More than books, food is incredibly personal. It's vital to our existence, it gives us life, and when we take it in, it becomes an intimate part of us and physically forms who we are and who we will become.

At the grocery store, I have a nosy habit of checking out what's going down the conveyor belt ahead of my own groceries. I like to look at the other customer's ingredients and imagine what he might be cooking with several pounds of carrots, flour, and onions. Such nosiness can result in a pretty intimate look into their lives, like if they are on a diet, are planning a party, own a cat, or just had a baby. What we have on the grocery conveyor belt or in our fridge is more revealing than what is on our bookshelves. For one thing, it's much more honest. Considering my bookshelf, there are books there I've read, but there are also books I haven't read, and as a way

---

3. "Foodie" is annoying and twee, but "gourmand" makes you sound about 800 pounds; "epicure" has a sterile, scientific ring to it; and "gastronome" sounds like a farting Hobbit. I personally prefer "glutton," because it's all encompassing: I'm not just into the "right" foods but also the "wrong."

to cloud the issue even more, there are books I've read, didn't like, but still shelve. That wouldn't happen in your fridge. You wouldn't keep something in your fridge that you ate and didn't like. You'd toss it. In many ways, bookshelves can be outright deceitful. While there are some people like my friend Meghan, who says she uses her bookshelves as a "record of [her] intellectual microhistory," there are others like Gloria Upson, the *Auntie Mame* character, who says, "Books are awfully decorative, don't you think?" Sometimes books are just window dressing—there because they look good or complement a color scheme.

Books tell you a person's interests; fridges tell you who they are.

The intimate connection we have with food is what builds community and brings people together. When there's a new baby or a new neighbor, people bring food. When there's a death or a natural disaster, people bring food. Food is essential to life, and we eat three times (or more, I'm not judging) a day. So yeah, we will die without food, but that doesn't necessarily explain why we get so emotional and judgmental over *other* people's food choices.

Katie Lambert, a former picky eater turned foodie, admits to me that she can get really angry when people won't try a particular food. "And I catch myself getting really heated up about it. It's like, why am I so invested in whether or not *she* tries something?" Katie wonders. Well, if we were to get on the therapist's couch about it, rejecting the offer of food can be seen as a rejection of the person offering the food or even a rejection of love. Think about experiencing a wonderful bite of pizza with a sauce that tastes like nothing you've ever had in this world. You're in fat, gustatory heaven and you want the person next to you—husband, wife, sister, kid, friend, mother—to have that same amazing experience because you love them, so you offer to share that experience with them. But they decline. In some sense, you might feel that they aren't just rejecting your offer of a shared experience; they are rejecting *you*.

Equalizing food with love is actually something parents are warned about in children's feeding books. If your baby, toddler, child, etc., doesn't want to eat the food you made for them, do not see it as a rejection of love. That's not what it's about for them, and it's certainly not what it's about for picky eaters. In fact, it's the reverse. *Not* forcing me to eat this food means you love me. It means you understand and respect my boundaries.

Melissa, who is a serious foodie married to someone who really doesn't like food, has never taken her husband's refusal to eat her food as a rejection. However, she admits, "It's hard for me because I am a true textbook extrovert and the primary characteristic of a textbook extrovert is the need to share the things they love with the people they love." Melissa gets most frustrated when her husband is sick, because she can't dose him up with her matzo ball soup. "That's the only way we know how to fix things [in my family]. Someone's not feeling well, you make them matzo ball soup. Someone lost a parent, you went over with a kugel. We fix things with food; that's how I was born and raised." Melissa explains that being unable to take care of her husband bothers her far more than it bothers him. He tells her that just her being there with him is taking care of him.

Melissa's husband was an Honest Picky Eater from the beginning, and she never saw it as a detraction even early in their dating years. "Because he was just so interesting!" Melissa tells me. They were open and honest in their communication about his picky eating, and as a result, Melissa always figured that there would be a way for them to navigate around it. Because food is such a major part of Melissa's life and one that she can't share with her husband, Melissa does what Amy Sargent, a licensed marriage and family therapist, counsels her clients to do in similar situations: She explores that part of her life with other people. She goes out to dinner with a group of girlfriends whose only rule is that they have to eat at a new restaurant, she and another foodie friend take and coteach cooking classes, and she gives huge dinner parties where she can make all the food she wants and be assured that it will be eaten and enjoyed by someone. The time she spends with her husband is focused on doing things they both like to do—volleyball, tennis, movies, reading, and being outdoors.

Melissa says what really unites them is their shared worldview. "We just maneuver through the world in the same way and that's what I want in a life partner, because I can always go to dinner with a girlfriend, but when I'm making life decisions, he's my sounding board for everything and he's the person that I trust more than anyone in the world." So while food is clearly important to Melissa, it's not the most important thing to them as a couple.

Coming up with other things to do as a couple can be a challenge since so much of what we do involves food, especially when it comes to celebrating important events such as anniversaries, birthdays, or work promotions. For a couple with food preference incompatibility, Amy suggests that these are the times to consider having a game night or going dancing, bowling, or miniature golfing—something where food is secondary and not the focus of the night. "Because it causes more stress and anxiety for the person who is not an adventurous eater, then they carry that into the relationship. And the other person, if they get frustrated, carries *that* into the relationship, so just because you want to have a pleasurable meal out, you're actually both getting some toxicity, which you're adding into the relationship," Amy explains.

An article in the *Washington Post* gave me serious pause about how other people deal with picky eaters in relationships. The article is about a woman named JoAnn whose then-boyfriend took her to Spain with a planned proposal in mind. However, once they got there and JoAnn "melted down" over a plate of paella, the trip went sour. According to the article, James Polickoski waited a year before he proposed and even then secured a promise from JoAnn that she would try all foods at least once. But JoAnn is an Honest Picky Eater. JoAnn had informed James that she couldn't eat things that had "head, bones or scales," so it's no wonder she flipped out when faced with paella containing heads-on crawfish.

I don't truly believe food alone breaks people up; it's more likely just a symptom that something else is wrong in the relationship. It could be that the picky eater really *is* narrow-minded or closed-off in all other parts of their life. Or it could mean the nonpicky eater—who always comes off seeming like the "right" one in these situations, for some reason—isn't equipped with enough compassion or patience to work within a picky eater's limitations.

For my friend Kira and for Katie Lambert, picky eating was not the main problem in past relationships, but both tell me that it would have been an ongoing issue if the relationships had continued. Kira, who lives and works in Southern California, felt the rigidity her picky eater ex-boyfriend exhibited in the food area mirrored rigidity in other parts of his life. "He could also be controlling, obsessive, and lacking in empathy," she adds. Interestingly, while the boyfriend ate a very narrow diet (starches, pizza, popcorn, and chicken), he didn't see himself as picky. Instead, he saw his way of eating as "correct," and anyone who ate differently from him was wrong.

And because the boyfriend didn't think there was anything wrong with the way he ate, Kira had the unfortunate task of running interference between him and their friends, which was very stressful for her and sometimes contentious. Most of their friends knew about the boyfriend's eating habits, but if a restaurant outing was proposed and the restaurant did not serve the "right" kind of food for the boyfriend, Kira would have to try and broker a deal. She would attempt to cajole the friends into going somewhere else—somewhere that was acceptable to the boyfriend—and sometimes it worked. Other times, their friends went to the new restaurant without them.

With Kira's boyfriend, there was no compromise, just a flat-out refusal to go somewhere new or eat something new. When the couple finally broke up, friends shook their heads over how Kira was able to stand the relationship as long as she did.

On the other hand, Katie, a web editor and freelance writer in Georgia, decided to go down the shaming route the first time she met her picky boyfriend in a group of friends. A group of them had dinner at a seafood restaurant perched on the edge of the ocean, and at this restaurant with the bounty of the sea at the doorstep, the boyfriend ordered chicken fingers. "I mocked him mercilessly," Katie says. "His palate is that of a five-year-old." Not embarrassed by his food choices, the boyfriend accepted the mocking with good humor, and they went on to date for five months. However, for Katie, his food choice was a red flag from the get-go. Not too much time would pass before she'd learn just how many "bizarre food phobias" he had, none of which made sense to her.

Katie says that if they had kept dating, his pickiness would have had a significant and adverse effect on the relationship. Katie, who had been fairly picky herself, is now a foodie. She eats at a wide variety of restaurants and is constantly challenging herself with new foods. Food has become a passion for her and it's important to her that she find someone with whom she can share this passion. Someone who is interested and informed enough to intelligently discuss food. The chicken-finger-eating boyfriend wasn't going to be that someone.

In Amy's opinion, the fact that Katie could forecast early on that the boyfriend's pickiness was going to become a major issue is really important. Amy, who has counseled couples who have dealt with food incompatibilities in their relationships, would applaud Katie for being able to identify her interest in food as a "value"—something that was very important to her—before the relationship went too much further. (Other values could be politics, religion, cats vs. dogs, starting a family, etc.) Amy explains, "If you're a real foodie and you love experiencing new foods, going to exotic places in the world and eating their dishes, then that's going to be a value you hold really high. Our culture does so much surrounding food that [identifying that value] is going to be in that person's benefit. If you are dating someone who will limit you, it's going to be a different kind of ball and chain."

It's understandable that if you want to live your life one way—eating at a lot of new restaurants, trying new foods, etc.—then being involved in a relationship that limits that could be very frustrating. Couples whose culinary incompatibility is an ongoing problem are constantly dealing with one half of the couple feeling pressured to eat things they can't eat and the other half of the couple feeling held back or restricted as a result. For the couple that cooks at home more than they eat out, the fights can build if one person is doing all the cooking and the other is doing all the food refusing. Or even more annoying, if separate meals have to be made just to accommodate both parties. All of this builds resentment on both sides of the couple.

Throwing kids into the mix results in yet another picky vs. nonpicky throw-down. Some people who don't want to be romantically involved with a picky eater say it's because they fear that a picky parent will beget picky children. To that I would counter, "Yeah, but they could get *your* nose!" Because, really, it's all a crapshoot with kids. Sure, picky eating *might* be hereditary and picky eating *might* come about if the kids imitate the picky parent (called "modeling" in science and child development circles), but it also might not happen at all.

When I ask Melissa how she feels about future children, she unsurprisingly says that she hopes they eat like her. Surprisingly, her husband hopes they eat like him. Because, Melissa explains, her husband feels that no one understood how he ate. As a kid, he was incredibly stubborn, and that stubbornness was a trait his parents didn't reckon on when he chose to spend the whole night at the dinner table rather than eat his dinner. Melissa says her husband will never force their children to eat anything.

Not forcing the food issue is key, not just in feeding kids, but in relationships as well. Before he was happily married, a friend of mine had a theory that people in relationships are waging a constant battle to change the other person. According to Russ, in this trench warfare, whoever changes the other person more wins. "I would say this about anything—not just about picky eating—you cannot change another person," Amy advises.

That's probably why it worked out for Mark and me. Mark would never pressure me to eat more than I wanted. He was never annoyed and would never make fun of me, criticize me, or make me feel as though my painful, shameful food aversions were doing something to him. He never tried to change me. Instead, because of his gentleness and kindness and enthusiasm for all new foods, I found myself wanting to try more things. I wanted to change, to be more like Mark, and as a result, I eventually transformed from a Lying Picky Eater to an Honest Picky Eater and then from picky eater to foodie. Mark helped this along without putting any pressure on me. He let me try things from his plate. He ordered things he thought I might like and cleaned off the things from my plate I didn't want.

Of course, if you were to ask him today, he'll say he was pretty clueless about my pickiness. "I definitely thought it wasn't possible to be allergic to peppers," he conceded recently. And the truth of it is, food wasn't all that important to Mark. He loves it, for sure, and his parents called him a "Professional Eater" when he was growing up, but he didn't define it as a value he prioritized in a relationship. Even if I had stayed picky, he would have still married me. Uh, that is, I *think* he would have still married me. One afternoon I ask him that very question. Mark slowly raises his eyes from his computer and looks steadily at me. "Yes," he says carefully.

It's true that I still draw a line at things he gulps down happily, but it's also true that my palate has progressed to the point where I now have my own vial of Lucianovic's Powdered Fire. I also do all the cooking because I learned that a picky eater who is in control of the kitchen is a happier picky eater.

CHAPTER 9

Picky Eater, Sleeping Foodie

Picky eaters don't pick off, scrape off, or "eat around" foreign objects. Take the basic example of a sandwich. If a picky eater likes a plain tuna sandwich with nothing added other than mayonnaise, don't give them tuna *salad* and shrug that they can just "pick out" or "eat around" the celery, pickles, capers, relish, or whatever other highfalutin ingredients you shoved in there. My childhood bologna sandwiches were bread, bologna, and French's yellow mustard. If my mother momentarily lost her head and tried to sneak in a layer of mayonnaise or a blandly innocent leaf of iceberg lettuce, that sandwich was trash-bound. And there was no sense in telling me I could just remove the lettuce and continue eating. I could still taste lettuce sweat on my bologna slice, and it was the taste of evil.[1]

Jess Thomson is someone I went to culinary school with,

1. It didn't matter that I'd eat iceberg lettuce in a salad. It didn't belong on a sandwich. Ever.

but I didn't know until recently that she is also a former picky eater. Jess tells me that one of the things she feared most was going out to dinner, specifically to McDonald's. She was afraid she wouldn't get her plain cheeseburger. "I was petrified that it wouldn't come plain, and that someone would suggest that I scrape things off. But don't they understand, *that's* not plain?" Jess demands, outraged. Why isn't scraping off good enough for a picky eater? "Because you don't want any microscopic evidence," Jess clarifies. Exactly. Picky eaters can taste the flavor watermark that every unwanted addition leaves on the surrounding food.

For years, I constantly wondered what was wrong with me. Why couldn't I just eat the way everyone else ate? None of my other friends could taste flavor watermarks. And no good telling me it's what made me "special," because every kid knows that "special" really means you're such a freak that they haven't invented an actual word for you yet. I thought I might be able explain it away by claiming supertaster status, but as my adventures in scientific experimentation reveal, that's a wash. But pawing through abstruse articles is about to pay off as science throws picky eaters another bone.

A 2008 article in the *British Journal of Nutrition* notes, "Many children also dislike foods with 'bits' or pips, the unexpected presence of which might signal contamination of some kind."

After reading that, I jump up and run down the hall to tell Mark. It explains so much about my picky past! It explains why I used to avoid chunky pasta sauce and why I went through a stage where none of my foods were allowed to touch—it was all a fear of contamination! "You didn't want your foods to touch?" Mark asks uneasily. (He's learning so much about me.) I ignore this and am off and babbling that my abhorrence of foods touching or being combined was because I instinctually believed that my food could be poisoned. "Poisoned?" Mark repeats, even more uneasily.

Did I truly believe my mother was trying to murder her second-born? Of course not; it was an unconscious, unrealized whatchamacallit—an instinct, I guess, buried deep down wherever instincts are buried. Using the fear of contamination revelation as a jumping-off point, maybe the picky eaters who are afraid to try new foods (food neophobes) are afraid because their instincts tell them to fear the unknown. Because there's every chance that the unknown could turn out to be poisonous, and eating indiscriminately has the potential to be deadly.

Maybe we, the picky, are more in touch with this cautious instinct compared to the rest of the population.

Maybe we, the picky, are the ones who said, "The Borgias invited us over for another wine and cheese tasting? Tell them we're busy."

Maybe we, the picky, are next in line to evolve to a higher plane of existence. Like Obi-Wan Kenobi, if a sodden pile of succotash tries to strike me down, I shall become more powerful than you could possibly imagine.

The best part about picky eaters evolving above and beyond everyone else is how far in the future higher planes of existence tend to be, so no one can prove we aren't on track to do just that.

While at Monell's DNA Camp, I float this theory to Dr. Reed. Might picky eaters be the ultimate survivors? "Yes," Dani responds, "but they will also starve to death in times of famine." Yeah, there is that little issue, I guess. Dani tells me about some Scandinavian farmers who colonized Greenland in the tenth century. The explorers brought sheep and dairy cows with them,

but after a few rough winters and a dearth of nourishing vege-
tation, the farmers were forced to slaughter and live off their
cattle and hunting dogs. Once those food sources were gone,
some archaeologists hypothesize, the colonists had nothing left
to eat. Greenland's waters would have been teeming with fish
and seal, but since the farmers refused, for whatever reason, to
learn how to fish, the colony was completely wiped out by 1500.[2]

Fine, so maybe we aren't more highly evolved, but you
probably won't catch a picky eater playing Russian roulette
with their life by ordering fugu at a sushi bar.

Fugu, the Japanese word for blowfish, is a great delicacy
in Japan. But there's a catch: It also contains a neurotoxin
called tetrodotoxin, which cannot be destroyed by cooking
and is 275 times deadlier than cyanide. The highest concentration of the neurotoxin lurks in the fugu's roe, ovaries, and
liver, but smaller amounts can also be found skulking in the
intestines, skin, and—in some species—the muscle tissue.
(That last disturbs me the most, since muscle tissue is the
main part of the fish that we eat.)

Captain Cook, who, along with two of his naturalists, came
uncomfortably close to dying from blowfish poisoning while
discovering New Caledonia in 1774, offers a vivid description
of his ordeal via his captain's logs from the HMS *Resolution*:

> We were seized with an extraordinary weakness
> all over our limbs attended with a numbness or
> sensation like to that caused by exposing ones

---

2. New and groundbreaking theory about the Lost Colony of Roanoke: They
were picky eaters who gagged "CROATOAN" at the idea of eating barbecue.

hands or feet to a fire after having been pinched
by much frost, I had almost lost the sence of feeling nor could I distinguish between light and
heavy bodies, a quart pot full of Water and a fea-
ther was the same in my hand.

After Cook and his naturalists "took a Vomet" and sweated
a bunch, they recovered from their blowfish bout. Sadly, a
shipboard pig, who snacked on the residual guts, was not as
lucky.[3]

If not prepared correctly—and the training to learn how
to do this is rigorous—the meat of the fish could be contaminated and deadly. This is such serious food prep that there
are laws in Japan governing it. Chefs undergo training to learn
the ways of the fugu, and only those who pass all their tests
are allowed to touch it.

"Even so," *The Oxford Companion to Food* warns, "instances
occur of Japanese dying from fugu poisoning, *usually* because
someone without the necessary skill has attempted to prepare
the fish." (Emphasis mine, because it freaks me out.) My point
is, people have died, and I'm willing to bet none of them were
picky eaters, and I'm just saying if that isn't Darwinism, I
don't know what is.

Okay, so maybe it isn't Darwinism, but it certainly speaks

---

3. A historian's footnote on this particular log entry noted that naturalist
Johann Forster's detailing of the event was slightly different. Apparently,
Forster thought that the fish might be poisonous, citing its ugly shape and
largeness of head, and told the good captain they should be wary of it. However, Captain Cook, who, the footnote said, was "stubborn about food,"
insisted he had eaten this fish before and been totally fine.

to the idea that picky eaters are very careful about what they eat. Who else is careful about what they eat? Foodies.

Chefs, gourmands, and foodies around the world are fond of telling anyone with half an ear that we taste first with our eyes and then with our mouths. It is no different for a picky eater. In fact, to a picky eater, presentation is of supreme importance.

Let's revisit the humble sandwich example. A sandwich's presentation relies primarily on the way it is cut. This is very important. A whole sandwich is wholly unappealing—who wants to gnaw their way through acres of thick crust just to get to the sweetest, tenderest part of the sandwich, i.e., the middle? Unthinkable. The sandwich has to come in two or four pieces to be palatable.

As a kid, you either got four squares or four isosceles triangles. I ask Joyce Slaton (former picky eater turned foodie) if she had an opinion on sandwich shapes. "Oh, triangles!" Joyce answers immediately. "It didn't taste right any other way. If you cut it into four little squares instead of triangles, they're more crusty on the edge. It's wrong if you cut it any other way." She's right, you know; triangles have a way more acceptable bread-to-crust ratio. I ask Joyce what she thought was so wrong with crusts. "It's the texture." The crusts are dryer and tougher than the rest of the sandwich, and the sandwich fixings never manage to spread far enough to the sandwich's perimeter to make sure the crusts taste like anything other than crusts. As a kid, Joyce also firmly believed that eating chicken noodle soup out of a thermos was a very important component of her lunch, but not just any thermos would do. It had to be her red thermos. Why? Because, Joyce tells me, "It tasted better that way."

In studying food neophobia in children, some folks in the

science community have determined that "foods that do not 'look right' to the child will be initially rejected based on vision alone." I'd like to note here that even as an adult who thinks I've put most of my picky past behind me, foods that don't please my eye will probably not please my palate. Now, does that sound picky or does that sound foodie? Dr. Nancy Zucker at Duke doesn't necessarily think there's a distinction between the two.

During our conversation, I tell Dr. Zucker I believe my conversion to being a foodie is a direct result of having been a picky eater for so many years, and that it is the same for other pickies turned foodies I know. Perhaps the intensity with which you hate certain foods is directly related to how much you will love them once you get over that first hump of trying them and discovering you actually really like them. It's as if the emotion and the energy are refocused. My friend Jane said it best when she told me that when she finally opened herself up to trying new and delicious foods, her world "went from black and white to Technicolor." It turned her from a picky eater to a full-blown foodie.

Dr. Zucker responds, "I think that's a great theory. I think another equally compatible theory is that being a foodie is a socially sanctioned way to be picky . . . because foodies are picky! But it's based on refinement and taste, right? For a foodie, there is this rapturous love of food, but there's also this demand for quality and so [they] can say as a foodie, 'Oh, I really prefer this specific kind of bread because it's really crusty and fresh out of the oven and I really don't prefer this other kind of bread, it tastes a little old to me, a little stale.' And I'm not being 'picky' because I'm really appreciating the sensual qualities of the food—well, that's what a picky eater is!"

In the *When Harry Met Sally* parlance, a picky eater (and

a foodie) just wants their food the way they want it. Going back to my sandwich example, I ask Joyce if she had a jam versus jelly opinion when she was a PB&J-eating kid. "No lumps! Had to be jelly! No fucking jam with those gross lumps—are you kidding me?" Joyce retorts. (Picky-eaters-turned-foodies are nothing if not opinionated.) Today, Joyce cans her own jelly and processes it exactly the way she likes it. Just like I'll cook certain vegetables the way I like them and don't really enjoy eating them any other way.

In a *Fresh Air* interview on National Public Radio, acclaimed food writer Ruth Reichl talked about learning to cook as a defensive strategy. To protect herself from being served the bizarre combinations her mother dreamed up—beef with chocolate sauce and half an apple pie added to a stew are just two examples—Reichl took over in the kitchen. While Reichl was not a picky eater herself, the idea of playing defense in the kitchen and needing to control what or how something is cooked is one picky eaters can understand.

England-born Samantha (Sam) Breach might be one of the most accomplished cooks I know. When she gives elaborate, multicourse dinner parties in her San Francisco loft apartment, the cupboards in her open kitchen are covered with multicolored sticky notes that meticulously map out every step and each task of her entire cooking process. Her love for food and cooking is so inexhaustible that part of a plan to thwart potential jet lag before flying home to England was, she Tweeted, to "wake up to a midnight feast of bacon and gougères." *Gougères* are a savory, Gruyère cheese-lacquered pastry made from the same dough (called *choux* paste or *pâté à choux*) that also produces beignets, éclairs, and cream puffs. Requiring a piping bag, a special nonstick baking surface called a Silpat, and a gentle touch, preparing these light, empyrean bites of cheese puffiness is no trifling task. Some people would never even attempt them, and others would be certainly disinclined to make them in the middle of the night and would perhaps instead rely on something easier or faster as part of a jet lag–thwarting plan. But not Sam. Sam got up and made gougères at midnight and "lunched" on them at 4 a.m. as she kept pushing herself into Greenwich mean time. It was a shock to my system to learn that Sam became such an accomplished, driven cook because she was a picky eater.

Sam's method for hiding food, which she called "pouching," was unlike anything I had ever tried as a kid. She stuffed unwanted food inside her cheeks and below her gum line, where it was out of sight, and she held it there, even while continuing to eat and swallow other food she could handle, until she could secretly get rid of the food by spitting it out. "I hated food," Sam says. Sam's family wasn't wealthy, so they grew a lot of their own vegetables and procured the cheapest cuts of meat. They derived no pleasure from eating. "Postwar Britain hadn't got the memo telling them they were allowed to enjoy food again," Sam says about growing up in Bristol in the late sixties and early seventies. Sam ate a lot of overcooked vegetables and tough, chewy meat. "Let's just face it, my mum really didn't know that much about cooking." Sam's mother, who was a single parent for many years and worked hard to give her two daughters the best she could manage, viewed food simply as fuel and didn't enjoy preparing it. "Because she didn't like cooking, she always encouraged my interest in it."

Sam suspects her early interest in cooking was based on

"an inner belief that food experiences could be better" if she were the one doing the cooking. Little by little, Sam learned to cook a few things—roast chicken and a perfect cheese sauce to serve with cauliflower—but most of her early forays in the kitchen were driven by what drives a lot of kids—her sweet tooth—so she became the family baker. Then, in her teens, Sam fell hard for mushrooms. "Instead of spending my pocket money on sweets, I would go to the greengrocer's and buy a quarter pound of mushrooms, take them home, and fry them up for a snack," Sam says. "I was beginning to learn that if only *I* could control what I ate instead of someone else controlling what I ate, then maybe it wouldn't be so bad after all." When she left home and was finally fully in control of whatever went in her mouth, Sam made a deal with herself: "I promised myself only delicious things would go there . . . I wanted to cook everything."

Getting better at and enjoying the cooking process was a major factor in getting past my own picky predilections. Once it became obvious that an editorial assistant's wages could not support how often I ate out in Boston, I tried to reproduce restaurant meals at home. Even as a kid, I enjoyed cooking and got multiple opportunities to do it when my mom went out of town. Now, it is true that I burned quite a few pans of rice and that I ruined my family's microwave when I thought I could make toast in it, but those catastrophes never stopped me from trying again. I even invented my own recipes. Well, I invented *one* recipe. It was called "Butter Soup" and consisted entirely of a large mass of melted butter with some scallions added in for seasoning. (You have to understand, I really loved butter as a kid. I still do, I just don't think I would, you know, *drink* it again.) It was a huge disappointment mostly because it was a bit weird to swallow all that butter. As it went down, it sort of coated and stuck oddly to my throat. That was the last time I made that particular recipe.

Experimenting aside, another reason I loved cooking for my family was because of the control I wielded. When I was in charge, we were going to eat what I liked. And if that meant corn or artichokes were the only vegetables we had for five days straight, so be it. As an adult cooking for myself, I reveled in that same control but the difference was, the more I cooked as an adult, the more new foods I tried. Once I started opening myself up to foods I thought I hated only to discover I actually liked them, it made me want to see if that was true for even more foods. That interest in new foods led to an interest in learning everything I could about cooking and food. At the time, I was an assistant editor at a fine arts and photography imprint at a large publishing company. It's not that I didn't enjoy working on seventy-five-dollar coffee-table books of famous photographers, but the more I immersed myself in food and cooking at home, the more I wanted to be a cookbook editor or a food writer for the rest of my life. When the publishing company moved all of editorial to the New York office, I took my severance to culinary school.

I never wanted to work in a professional kitchen. At thirty years old, I knew I didn't have the stamina for the job or the tolerance for the machismo I had read so much about in Anthony Bourdain's *Kitchen Confidential*, but I did think culinary school would give me the food background I needed to pursue a career in food writing or editing. While at culinary school, I learned a lot of things. I learned I could be on my feet for eight hours as long as I wore clogs, I learned that burns were a badge of honor but cuts were a mark of stupidity, and of course, I learned a lot about food and how to cook it. However, the most important thing I took away from culinary school was how to season properly.

Tasting as you cook is the only way to know if the seasoning of a dish is correct. *In your opinion.* Remember how Dr. Zucker and I said in Chapter 6 that no one can understand what is going on in a person's mouth? That's why tasting as you go is the best way to judge if food is seasoned to your liking. Not the recipe's liking, that's just a guide, but *your* liking. I started calling the director of my culinary school "the Salt Monster" because after tasting everyone's finished dishes, she always proclaimed: "Needs more salt." This boggled us because, after all, we were following *her* recipes to the letter, so if the dish needed more salt, why didn't she reflect that in the ingredients? She was teaching us that recipes are just the starting point, and that we had to taste as we cooked to know when a dish had enough flavor.

Learning to cook doesn't just teach you about what tastes good and why, but it also demystifies food. My friend Anita—formerly picky turned foodie—had a lot of trouble eating ribs, chicken wings, "or anything on the bone that was recognizably an animal part" until she took a required butchery course at culinary school. After she learned how to break down poultry, pigs, and beef, Anita got past her squeamishness and was more willing to eat recognizable animal parts. "I'm sure some of it was just desensitization to an unpleasant thing through repeated exposure," Anita explains, "but I did really feel like learning the puzzle of how animals were put together—and I guess more to the point, taken apart—was a large part of being more comfortable in my place as a carnivore." So comfortable, in fact, that Anita now eats oxtail and bone marrow and roasts whole pigs in her backyard with her husband. It harks back to Dr. Zucker's belief that seeing the food in a different context—one that isn't a threatening context—can help reduce a picky eater's fear surrounding that food. Furthermore, if you can alter that context even more and morph your perception to the point where you start to actually enjoy certain aspects of food—like cooking it—it changes those set neural pathways even more dramatically.

Changing those neural pathways and associations is why parents of picky children are encouraged to bring them into the kitchen and cook with them in the hopes of broadening their palates. By doing this, not only are the kids gradually lowering their resistance to the food by participating in a fun activity with their parents, but they also develop a sense of ownership and pride in the task and become invested in the results of their labors. With this investment exists the potential for the kids to actually go so far as to taste the food they made, since the food is now associated with a pleasant experience rather than being seen as gross or bad.

This is not the case with all picky eaters, but I do think that so many picky eaters have had repeated bad experiences with food because the food was just bad. Not tasty, not at its best. While she didn't necessarily search for the perfect recipe to cook at home the way I did, Amy Watts still took a foodie approach to overcoming her food hates and decided that the way to force herself to like a food was to have it from her local James Beard–nominated chef. She said to herself, "This guy is a really good chef, so if he wants to serve me lentils, they're probably going to be damn good lentils." Amy was searching for the "platonic ideal" of foods when she decided to eat them for the first time. "So, in other words," she explains, "the first time I eat green beans, it isn't going to be a tin of Bush's from the Kroger. It's going to be haricots verts in a sherry reduction, or whatever." Properly cooked and seasoned food can make or break it for a picky eater.

It seems to be true in my case. All it took was finding that perfect recipe to change my impression of a hated food. Now there are some cases where I will eat a certain vegetable only one way, like how I'll eat okra only if it's sautéed the way my friend Catherine sautéed it, but other times one good encounter with a vegetable bolsters me enough to try another recipe. That happened with Brussels sprouts.

One day, I randomly decided to like Brussels sprouts. I tried them steamed once and agreed with almost everyone else on the planet that they were the most disgusting vegetable ever grown. However, after living in California for a few months and seeing the tight round balls mounded up at the farmers' market, I started craving them. Or since I already despised them, maybe what I was really craving was the *idea* of liking them. They looked so lovely in their green piles, so robust, and so full of healthful antioxidants. (I had recently reached an age where the thought of healthful food was way more appealing than it was off-putting.) I put out a call on my blog, "The Grub Report," for the best Brussels sprouts recipes my readers could offer. There was one caveat: no recipes that called for drowning the vegetable in flavor-deadening cheese sauce. I wanted to like Brussels sprouts for what they were, not for what they were smothered in.

The recipe that converted me, which called for roasting

them after they were marinated in balsamic vinegar, gave me the courage to try Alice Waters's method of sautéing the individually peeled-off leaves with garlic and hot pepper flakes. Between the two methods, I became Brussels sprouts obsessed. There's a theory among infant sleep experts that if a baby naps well, he will also sleep well at night. "Sleep begets sleep," they preach. I have started to apply that theory to overcoming picky eating. If a picky eater can transform just one food hate into a food like, it gives them the courage and impetus to try transforming other foods hates—food begets food.

After my Brussels sprouts experience, I realized that when it came to certain vegetables—the bane of my existence—it just took me having them the "right" way to like them, which started with finding the "right" cooking process. Usually it was roasting that brought out the best in vegetables, probably because the high heat brings all that wonderful caramelization to the surface of otherwise stenchy vegetables, such as cauliflower and broccoli. Food scientist Harold McGee explains, "Dry heating methods can dry out food surfaces and turn them crisp and brown. Dryness and high temperatures encourage food proteins and sugars to react with each other and form brown pigments and distinctive, rich flavors. Moist heating methods generally don't encourage these browning reactions, and don't develop the same richness of flavor." In the specific case of broccoli, which can taste bitter to some people or simply bland to others, Alton Brown explained on his show *Good Eats* that bringing out the natural sugars in broccoli counteracts the bitterness. I've never detected broccoli's bitterness, but the roasting process lends a deeper, richer flavor to what has always been a tasteless vegetable to me.

Other times, what worked was sautéing the vegetables so hot and so fast that they got fully cooked without breaking down into piles of green mush, losing all their flavor in a long cooking process. Sautéing, like roasting, is another method known as "dry heat cooking." "Moist heat cooking" are methods such as steaming, braising, and boiling. If you're very careful with your sauté and don't leave your vegetables in the pan to burn up, you can get some caramelization on the vegetables. However, for even caramelization with vegetables such as cauliflower, Brussels sprouts, or broccoli, I go for the low-maintenance oven roast.

(I was disabused of the notion that roasting improves any and all vegetables when I tried to roast bitter endive. That is one vegetable whose natural sugars are *not* able to counteract the bitterness just from a dry heat process. In fact, I've heard that the best recipe for endive is famed food writer Richard Olney's recipe that calls for braising the endive very slowly and very decadently with ham, butter, and cream.)

What I like about sautéing certain vegetables is the control it gives you. You are standing right there, moving your okra, greens, or Brussels sprout leaves around with tongs, and you see exactly when you want to pull the pan from the heat. Maybe you want to pull it just as the leaves on the beet greens start to wilt, or maybe you want to keep it on longer until the hardier rapini greens cook down more. Maybe you want a few leaves of the Brussels sprouts to brown a bit. It's all in your control.

I generally follow two rules when it comes to cooking vegetables: (1) Never steam or boil (I even oven-roast ears of corn now), and (2) never frozen or canned. The vegetables have to be fresh.

The only exceptions to those rules are dry legumes, such as shell beans and lentils, which actually have to be steamed or simmered; there's no way around it. And this brings us to finding the "right" recipe, because learning how to cook the food is only half the battle. Finding the right recipe—as in, figuring out what ingredients you want to add to that cooked food—is what will carry you to gustatory victory. I did find that some foods, such as roasted cauliflower, were amazing with just three ingredients—olive oil, salt, and pepper—yet others required more enhancements to make me actually enjoy eating them.

Get sauced

After trying to enjoy lentils and shell beans as the purists recommended—with just olive oil, salt, and pepper—and having all the flavor sucked out of my mouth, I relaxed my "no cheese sauce" rule and started jazzing them up with sauces and vinaigrettes. My favorite lentil recipe calls for presteamed lentils from Trader Joe's to be folded into a garlicky, Dijon mustard–based vinaigrette, which is then accented with olives, sliced celery, and chopped parsley. With shell beans, I tend to go for a hearty, homemade marinara or Bolognese sauce, to which I'll often add sautéed greens. I treat lentils and shell beans as if they were a pasta or a salad and develop recipe ideas from that starting point.

If you don't like the texture or flavor of something, change it

I can't stand the sweetness or mushiness of squash, sweet potatoes, and yams. However, instead of depriving my body of all the good stuff that comes from eating orange fruits and roots, I came up with ways to overcome their sweetness with savory.[4] With butternut squash, I roasted it until it was soft enough that I could use a fork to mash in some minced garlic, scallions, and red pepper flakes. To deal with its mushy texture and to continue upping the savory quotient, I used the mashed squash as a "sauce" to coat blue cheese–stuffed tortellini. Combining a previously hated food with pasta was also a way to change its texture and dilute its flavor a bit. To downplay their flavor impact, I mixed every vegetable I was trying to like with cooked pasta and topped the whole thing off with grated cheese. It's actually a work-around I rely on to this day when eating greens.

As I've probably made clear, I don't like big piles of cooked greens, because their slimy and hard-to-chew texture prods my gag reflex into action. It helps to break up the greens with a different texture—one that comes from pasta, farro, or shell beans. (Also, scads of garlic and snowy drifts of freshly grated Parmigiano-Reggiano or Pecorino never hurt.)

Watching famously picky eater Anderson Cooper try spinach on TV recently, I cringed because it looked like he'd forked up a bite of plain, sautéed spinach. (Anderson, honey, there's no need to do that to yourself. Let me cook greens for you.) After all, where's the rule that says you have to eat vegetables as plain as possible? Adding ingredients you actually like to

---

4. Orange vegetables, fruits, and roots contain vitamins A and C primarily, but also iron and riboflavin. Sweet potatoes are a superfood, and the general rule of thumb is, the more colorful your plate, the healthier your body.

something you don't like is a way to change your negative associations with that food. I sincerely believe that, in many cases, it just takes finding the right recipe to turn a broccoli/spinach/Brussels sprouts hater into a broccoli/spinach/Brussels sprouts lover.

Vegetables: Recipes to Love By

So much do I love my carefully studied ways of doing up certain vegetables that I won't eat them at restaurants if I think they are cooked "wrong." If that sounds a bit controlling, well, then maybe there is something in the idea that picky eaters and OCD sufferers have something in common. Frankly, I don't really care how it makes me sound; I've finally found ways to love certain vegetables so much that they, rather than the meat, end up being the star of the meal. But you don't have to take my word for it; I've converted quite a few people with the following recipes.

ROASTED BRUSSELS SPROUTS

I recently tried the aforementioned sauté recipe on company, but instead of serving with pasta, as Alice suggests in her cookbook, I served the sautéed leaves as a salad with apples. I got an email from one of my guests saying that she normally doesn't like Brussels sprouts, but she had two helpings that night. However, this roasting technique is the original recipe that opened my mouth to the deliciousness that is the Brussels sprout.

Hat tip to TC Duong, the originator of this recipe.

4 tablespoons olive oil
3 tablespoons balsamic vinegar
2-3 cloves minced garlic
1 teaspoon salt
1 teaspoon freshly ground black pepper
1 pound Brussels sprouts, trimmed of blemished outer leaves
    and halved

Preheat oven to 425°.

1. In a large bowl, whisk the olive oil, vinegar, garlic, salt, and pepper together. Add the Brussels sprouts to the marinade, toss to coat with the marinade, and let sit for 5–10 minutes.

2. Spread the Brussels sprouts evenly out on a roasting pan and roast for 15–20 minutes or until the sprouts are tender and caramelized.

ROASTED CAULIFLOWER

Roasting up cauliflower was another revelation. "It's like McDonald's french fries without the guilt!" Mark told me on night three of our All Cauliflower All the Time diet.

1 head cauliflower
2-3 tablespoons olive oil
1-2 teaspoons salt
1-2 teaspoons freshly ground black pepper

Preheat the oven to 500°.

1. Break apart or cut the cauliflower into florets.

2. In a large bowl, toss the florets with olive oil until coated and glistening. Add the salt and pepper and toss again.

3. Scatter the florets on a cookie sheet or roasting pan with low sides and roast until the cauliflower becomes brown, about 30 minutes. Make sure to stir the cauliflower florets about halfway through to prevent burning and sticking.

SAUTÉED GREENS

The most ringing endorsement I have for this recipe is that I used it to convert twin picky eaters in a single day. (You could even say I ran my own twin study right out of my kitchen![5]) While it's true that Courtney was pretty brave when it came to trying foods, Keely—who got freaked out

---

5. Because of their shared genetic makeup and upbringing, scientists rely heavily on studies conducted on twins when trying to figure out if behavioral traits are influenced by environment or if they are hereditary. The "nature vs. nurture" debate is one area of study.

just talking to me about her greens and lettuce aversion—was the tougher nut to crack. And yet when she walked away from my table, she'd not just tolerated the greens I made, but had asked for seconds and had painstakingly transcribed the recipe. I also managed to get her to like certain lettuces by making her homemade vinaigrette using my very best olive oil.

You can always add your own twist to greens, like spicy sausage or tomato sauce with the greens and pasta or bacon with, well, pretty much everything.

4–5 ounces penne rigate pasta
1–2 tablespoons olive oil (the best you have)
8 cups greens, washed and chopped or torn into small pieces
    (start with the mildest greens, beet greens, and work your
    way up to chard and other stronger, heartier greens)
Salt, to taste
Freshly ground black pepper, to taste
Pinch red pepper flakes, optional
1–2 cloves minced garlic
¼ cup freshly grated Parmigiano-Reggiano (more if you want)

1. Fill three-quarters of a stockpot with water and bring it to a boil. Add one or two large pinches of salt to the water and then add the pasta. Cook according to box directions, usually 12–13 minutes.

2. While the pasta is cooking, warm the olive oil in a large skillet over medium-high heat, add the greens, and use tongs to stir the greens until they wilt. Add the salt and pepper and continue

stirring for another 1-2 minutes. Keep the greens on the heat longer if you want them to wilt more.

3. Take the skillet off the heat and add the red pepper flakes and the garlic. Stir until fully incorporated, allowing the residual heat of the greens to cook the garlic without burning it bitter.

4. Drain the pasta, add a splash of olive oil, stir, and put back in the pasta pot. Add the sautéed greens and cheese, and stir. Taste the pasta; if you don't think there's enough flavor, add more salt or cheese.

✕ ROASTED BROCCOLI WITH SMOKED ✕ PAPRIKA-SHERRY VINAIGRETTE

Within the last year, broccoli—of all things—has replaced corn as my comfort vegetable. Roasted broccoli, that is. It must always be roasted and, if possible, dressed with a smoked paprika vinaigrette, a genius recipe I found on Amanda Hesser and Merrill Stubbs's crowd-sourced recipe website Food52. This life-changing recipe, with minor changes by me, was contributed by Food52 participant arielleclementine.

For the broccoli
1-2 crowns broccoli, divided into florets
2 tablespoons olive oil
1-2 teaspoons salt

For the smoked paprika vinaigrette
   ¼ cup olive oil
   1 teaspoon smoked paprika
   2-3 cloves garlic, minced
   1½ tablespoons sherry vinegar
   ½ teaspoon salt

Preheat oven to 425°.

1. Toss the broccoli with the olive oil and salt, and spread out on a cookie sheet or roasting pan. Roast for 20 minutes.

2. While the broccoli is roasting, add the olive oil to a skillet and warm over medium heat for 1-2 minutes. Add the smoked paprika and garlic and remove from heat. Stir and set aside.

3. Add the sherry vinegar and salt to a small bowl and whisk in the smoked paprika and garlic oil.

4. In a large bowl, toss the roasted broccoli with 2 tablespoons of the smoked paprika vinaigrette and serve warm.

SAUTÉED OKRA

This recipe is based on the one my friend Catherine published on her food blog, "Food Musings," and is what she made the night I got addicted to okra.

2 tablespoons olive oil
1/2 pound okra, sliced into 1/4- or 1/2-inch pieces
2 teaspoons salt, to start with

1. Warm the oil in a large skillet over medium-high heat. Add the okra and cook, stirring frequently, for about 10–15 minutes. Catherine's recipe says to cook "until somewhat softened on the inside, crispy on the outside, and darkened to a deep green," and I like to cook until some pieces get slightly brown about the edges.

2. Add the salt, taste, and add more salt if so desired.

*

Digging up so many other cases of former picky eaters who, just like me, morphed into foodies was a complete surprise. Until I started asking around, I had no idea that some of the most ravenous food lovers I knew—Sam, who makes gougères at midnight; Anita, who roasts pigs in her backyard; and Joyce, who makes her own jam—were former picky eaters. Then again, if you go by Dr. Zucker's theory that foodies are just socially acceptable picky eaters, maybe all these former picky eaters are *still* picky eaters; it's simply that their pickiness manifests itself in a different way.

There are surely plenty of picky eaters out there who would never think of themselves as foodies and would be shocked to have themselves lumped in with a group of oxtail-eating food lovers, and of course, that's not what Dr. Zucker is saying. Her point is not that picky eaters are foodies, but that foodies are picky eaters, because at some level, both groups are happiest (or feel least threatened) when eating within the confines of restrictions. They are entirely different restrictions, of course, since typically, the restrictions a picky eater feels forced into limits the variety of food she eats—say, refusing all vegetables and living on starches and some meats—whereas the restrictions a foodie imposes are more about getting what is thought to be the best flavor out of a lot of different foods (eating only locally grown food, grass-fed beef, or raw milk cheese, etc.). As Dr. Zucker said, what drives a foodie's choices is bedrocked in quality, refinement, and taste. That's how a foodie can be seen as picky.

The most significant difference between a picky eater and a foodie comes down to free will, because being a foodie is a deliberate choice and being a picky eater isn't. It is a choice to eat only bread baked fresh that morning and never darken McDonald's door. It is not a choice to gag over all green vegetables or dread eating at a restaurant or a friend's house. However, when you're one of the hybrids like me, a former picky eater turned foodie, where being a foodie isn't so much a choice as it is an imperative if you want to actually enjoy your food, the situation becomes even more complicated.

After experiencing both the best and the worst food has to offer and after living too long harboring anxieties or active dislikes of a great many foods, a picky-foodie can't go backward. A picky-foodie has spent so much time knowing the worst of food that the refusal to accept anything less than what is a self-determined "best" food is really not based on some snobby-sounding, elitist principle. A picky-foodie refuses to accept less because he simply cannot eat whatever that less is. It's like growing up in a leaky shack and then finally living in an opulent mansion for a time, only to be told that you have to give up that life and go back to living in the leaky shack. You already know what kind of wretched life awaits you in that leaky shack, and it's that foreknowledge that makes going back intolerable. Once a picky-foodie has turned his back on the Dark Side of foods, all he wants to do is continue to discover new wonderful foods, and he does this either by becoming incredibly adventurous with his choices, taking control of cooking, or simply finding new ways of giving old foods a makeover.

That said, being adventurous or learning to cook or finding the perfect recipe isn't always going to work. Some food aversions run too deep to be "cured" or are due to factors extending beyond the steamy reach of the kitchen. For my part, I will confess that while I now adore Brussels sprouts and broccoli, cauliflower and beets, greens, fish, peaches, and okra, I will still never—not ever—eat a speck of succotash.

Something to Chew On

Whenever I try to explain what it's like to go from picky to foodie, I flash back to the time I heard someone taking a glass-half-full approach to manic-depression. The point was made that the non-manic-depressives can't possibly ever understand the lowest lows a manic-depressive feels, but they also don't ever get to feel the highest highs. That pretty much describes how I feel about my picky past and foodie future. But without the lithium. See, only someone who hated food as much as I once did would be able to love food with the same level of intensity as I do now. It's not an exaggeration to say that every time I reversed the polarity of a food hate, a minor miracle exploded in my life.

Minor miracles aside, I will admit that my life probably would have been much easier and less anxiety-riddled if I hadn't been stuffing food behind books or hiding peas under my knife for twenty-seven years. Yet I can't overlook the fact that my picky past is directly responsible for turning me into someone who loved food so much that I had to make a career out of it.

If I had grown up clinging to an Italian grandmother's apron strings, being fed handmade pasta, and helping stir a fifteen-hour red sauce, maybe I would have loved any and all food my whole life. Maybe I still would have become a food writer and editor. Maybe. (After all, growing up in a foodie family isn't always a guarantee against being picky.) But if I had grown up with a deep love of all foods bred into me from the start, I wouldn't have the joy of discovering that love on my own. Becoming a food lover, that's all me. I did that. I own that, and it's something I worked at for a long time. In fact, it's something I continue to work at, because it was only last year that I found a broccoli recipe that replaced enmity with adoration. If I hadn't been a picky eater from the start, I wouldn't get to know the pure, transcendent joy of loving food the way I do now because I never would have experienced the disgust, the revulsion, or the unrelenting gagging. I didn't just "get over" my disgust, revulsion, or gagging either. I crave broccoli, I lust after okra, I *need* Brussels sprouts.

As to the eternal question of, "But *why* was I a picky eater?," who knows. It wasn't because I was a supertaster, but that's pretty much all I know. It was probably a combination of factors. It was growing up with frozen vegetables. It was eating fishy freshwater fish. It was living in Minnesota. It was fear of the unknown. It was minor childhood trauma. It's my biology. It was being the middle child. It was having brown hair. It was just me.

But it's not just me. I originally thought I would end this book by giving a little speech about how elite we all are. That we, the picky, are the few, the proud, who will stand together in a more perfect union against the world. The thing of it is, adult picky eaters are more common than I imagined. They might be former, recovering, or current, but there are a lot of us. And we get each other. We get what it's like to dread eating at friends' houses or at strange restaurants. We get why it's simply not possible to "just try" a bite of this or that and how hard that is to explain to people who *don't* get it. We get the shame or embarrassment of living with picky eating day in, day out and stressing out about why we can't just be like "everybody else." We get what it's like for food to be a bone of contention or a source of stress in a relationship or family. Honestly, as picky parents, we also might be marginally more successful about backing off from picky kids since we know exactly what our child is going through. Had I not been a picky eater, I'm sure I would still worry about parenting a picky eater because being worried is my default setting. However, I will say that while being a former picky eater—and writing a book about it—may make me, ah, *unusually* susceptible to that particular worry, it also makes me sympathetic.

But most of all, we get that it's not a personality defect that makes us picky; it's just who we are. And whatever the cause, it's not our fault or choice. Take comfort in the community of picky eaters and in knowing that you are not alone.

And remember—stand picky, stand proud.

RESOURCES

Informational Websites

23andMe
www.23andMe.com

The Food F.A.D. [Finicky Eating in Adults] Study
www.dukehealth.org/clinicaltrials/the_food_fad_study_finicky_eating
_in_adults

Human Sniffer
www.youtube.com/watch?v=TUNQFIqoN7g

Indigo Instruments
www.indigo.com/test-strips/taste-test-strips.html
www.indigo.com/test-strips/gph-test-strips/ptc-taste-test-strips.html

The Mayo Clinic
www.mayoclinic.com

The Taste Science Laboratory, Division of Nutritional Science, Cornell University
www.tastescience.com/abouttaste1.html

Umami Information Center
www.umamiinfo.com

Books and Articles

Ackerman, Diane, *A Natural History of the Senses*. Vintage Books, 1990.
Anderson, Mark, "Your DNA, Decoded." *Delta Sky Magazine*, August 2010.

Barclay, Eliza, "Why Bacon Is a Gateway to Meat for Vegetarians." NPR
.org, January 28, 2011. www.npr.org/blogs/health/2011/02/02/
133304206/why-bacon-is-a-gateway-to-meat-for-vegetarians.

Birch, L. L., L. Gunder, K. Grimm-Thomas, and D. G. Laing, "Infants'
Consumption of a New Food Enhances Acceptance of Similar Foods."
Appetite 30(3), 283–95, 1998.

Blakeslee, Albert F., "Demonstration of Differences Between
People in the Sense of Smell." *Scientific American Monthly* 41(1), 72–84,
1935.

Brown, Alton, "If It Ain't Broccoli, Don't Fix It." *Good Eats*, The Food
Network, 2007.

Bryson, Bill, *At Home: A Short History of Private Life.* Anchor, 2011.

Bufe, Bernd, Paul A. S. Breslin, Christina Kuhn, Danielle R. Reed, Chris-
topher D. Tharp, Jay P. Slack, Un-Kyung Kim, Dennis Drayna, and
Wolfgang Meyerhof, "The Molecular Basis of Individual Differences
in Phenylthiocarbamide and Propylthiouracil Bitterness Perception."
Current Biology 15(4), 322–27, February 22, 2005.

Cashdan, E., "Adaptiveness of Food Learning and Food Aversions in
Children." *Social Science Information* 37(4), 613–32, 1998.

Chast, Roz, "Bananas." *New Yorker*, November 8, 2010.

Crenson, Matthew, "23andMe Struts Its Stuff in NYC During Fashion
Week." Spittoon Blog, September 11, 2008. http://spittoon.23andme
.com/2008/09/11/23andme-struts-its-stuff-in-nyc-during-fashion-week.

Child, Lauren, *I Will Never Not Ever Eat a Tomato.* Candlewick, 2003.

Crumpacker, Bunny, *The Sex Life of Food.* Thomas Dunne Books, 2006.

Daughtridge, Mary Margaret, *SEALed with a Kiss.* Sourcebooks Casa-
blanca, 2008.

Davidson, Alan, *The Oxford Companion to Food.* Oxford University Press,
2006.

Dizik, Alina, "Béchamel, Not Bug Juice, Next to the Campfire." *Wall Street
Journal*, August 20, 2010.

Dovey, Terence M., Paul A. Staples, E. Leigh Gibson, and Jason C. G.
Halford, "Food Neophobia and 'Picky/Fussy' Eating in Children:
A Review." *Appetite* 50, 181–93, 2008.

Dunnan, Nancy, and Nancy Tuckerman, *The Amy Vanderbilt Complete
Book of Etiquette: Entirely Rewritten and Updated.* Doubleday, 1995.

Ephron, Nora, *Heartburn.* Vintage, 1996.

Ernsperger, Lori, and Tania Stegen-Hanson, *Finicky Eaters: What to Do
When Kids Won't Eat!* Future Horizons, 2005.

Friedman, Emily, "Picky Eaters: When Waffles and Fries Are All You
Eat." ABCNEWS.go.com, August 10, 2010.

Galloway, Amy T., Yoona Lee, and Leann L. Birch, "Predictors and Consequences of Food Pickiness in Young Girls." *Journal of the American Dietetic Association* 103(6), 692–98, 2003.

Glander, K. E., "The Impact of Plant Secondary Compounds on Primate Feeding Behavior." *Yearbook of Physical Anthropology* 25, 1–18, 1982.

Glass, Ira, "This American Life 182: Cringe." April 13, 2001. WBEZ Chicago Public Media, PRI.

Glendinning, John I., "Is the Bitter Rejection Response Always Adaptive?" *Physiology & Behavior* 56(6), 1217–27, 1994.

Goodman, Leah McGrath, "Married to the Google Billionaire." *Marie Claire*, May 10, 2010.

Groer, Annie, "The Picky Eater Files." *Washington Post*, September 26, 2006.

Grose, Jessica, "Foodie Death Sentence." Slate.com, October 25, 2011.

Hagerty, Barbara Bradley, "What You Need to Know About Hare Krishnas." NPR.org, May 22, 2008. www.npr.org/templates/story/story.php?storyId=90643796.

Harlan, Jack R., *Crops and Man*. American Society of Agronomy–Crop Science Society, 1992.

Hesser, Amanda, *Cooking for Mr. Latte*. W. W. Norton, 2003.

The Journals of Captain Cook II: The Voyage of the Resolution and Adventure, 1772–1775. Hakluyt Society, Boydell Press, 1999, p. 535.

Kennedy, John F. "Address on the Cuban Missile Crisis." October 22, 1962. www.fordham.edu/halsall/mod/1962kennedy-cuba.htm.

Leopold, A. Carl, and Robert Ardrey, "Toxic Substances in Plants: The Food Habits of Early Man." *Science* 176, 512–13, 1972.

Lynes, Russell, *The Domesticated Americans*. Harper & Row, 1963.

McBurney, D. H., and J. F. Gent, "On the Nature of Taste Qualities." *Psychological Bulletin* 86, 151–67, 1979.

McGee, Harold, "Cilantro Haters, It's Not Your Fault." *New York Times*, April 14, 2010.

——, *Keys to Good Cooking: A Guide to Making the Best of Foods and Recipes*. Penguin Press, 2010.

Milton, John, *The Riverside Milton*, ed. by Roy Flannagan. Houghton Mifflin, 1998.

Nahmad, Valerie, "Something Like Savory." August 8, 2008. Chow.com. www.chow.com/food-news/53446/something-like-savory.

Newman, Susan, "Beating the Biological Clock." *Psychology Today*, June 14, 2011.

Oz, Mehmet, "Why Do I Hate Vegetables? And What Should I Eat Instead?" *Esquire*, February 20, 2007. www.esquire.com/features/ask-dr-oz/ESQ0207veggies?click=pp.

——, and Michael Roizen, *You on a Diet*. Free Press, 2009.

Parker-Pope, Tara, "Even Top Chefs Have Picky Kids." NYTimes.com, February 19, 2009. http://well.blogs.nytimes/2009/02/19/even-top-chefs-have-picky-kids.

Pollan, Michael, "Our National Eating Disorder." *New York Times Magazine*, October 2004. http://michaelpollan.com/articles-archive/our-national-eating-disorder.

Pool, Daniel, *What Jane Austen Ate and Charles Dickens Knew*. Touchstone, 1994.

Pringle, Heather, "Death in Norse Greenland." *Science* 275, February 14, 1997.

Reed, Danielle R., "Birth of a New Breed of Supertaster." *Chemical Senses* 33(6), 489–91, June 18, 2008.

Rosed, P., M. Bundgaard, J. Fiske, and A. M. L. Pedersen, "The Use of Acupuncture in Controlling the Gag Reflex in Patients Requiring an Upper Alginate Impression: An Audit." *British Dental Journal* 201, 721–25, 2006.

Rösler, Alexander, Bettina Otto, Dagmar Schreiber-Dietrich, Helmuth Steinmetz, and Kirn R. Kessler, "Single-Needle Acupuncture Alleviates Gag Reflex During Transesophageal Echocardiography: A Blinded, Randomized, Controlled Pilot Trial." *Journal of Alternative and Complementary Medicine* 9(6), 847–49, 2003.

Sassone, Bob, "Are You a Supertaster or an Undertaster?" *Slashfood*,February 8, 2008. www.slashfood.com/2008/02/08/are-you-a-supertaster-or-an-undertaster.

Satter, Ellyn, *Child of Mine*. Bull Publishing, 2000.

Shattuck, Catherine, "Ode to a Vegetable." FoodMusings.com, March 27, 2005. http://foodmusings.typepad.com/food_musings/2005/03/ode_to_a_vegeta.html.

Slaton, Joyce, "My Picky Eater Stole My Smug." Babycenter.com, August 25, 2010.

——, "Picky Eater? Not Your Fault." Babycenter.com, August 24, 2010.

Tagliaferro, Linda, *The Complete Idiot's Guide to Decoding Your Genes*. Alpha, 1999.

Tavernise, Sabrina, "Census Data Reveals a Shift in Patterns of Childbearing." *New York Times*, May 9, 2011.

Trager, James, *The Food Chronology*. Owl Books, 1997.

Viorst, Judith, *Alexander and the Terrible, Horrible, No Good, Very Bad Day*. Aladdin Paperbacks, 1976.

Wang, Shirley, "No Age Limit on Picky Eating." *Wall Street Journal*, July 6, 2010.

Wardle, Jane, and Lucy Cooke. "Genetic and Environmental Determinants of Children's Food Preferences." *British Journal of Nutrition* 99, Suppl. 1, S15–S21, 2008.

Waters, Alice, *Chez Panisse Vegetables.* HarperCollins, 1996.

Wilson, Amy Lyles, *Cooking with Friends.* Rutledge Hill Press, November 1995.

Wurtman, Judith, and Nina Frusztajer Marquis, *The Serotonin Power Diet.* Rodale Books, 2006.

Press Releases

"Bitter Taste Identifies Poisons in Foods." Monell Chemical Senses Center Press Release, September 18, 2006.

"Children's Taste Sensitivity and Food Choices Influenced by Taste Gene." Monell Chemical Senses Center Press Release, February 7, 2005.

"Individual Differences in Taste Perception Directly Related to Genetically-Determined Variation in Taste Receptors." Monell Chemical Senses Center Press Release, February 21, 2005.

Online Sources

"Are You a Supertaster?" www.bbc.co.uk/science/humanbody/body/interactives/supertaster.

"Cultural Gaffes at Home and Abroad." Peace Corps. www.peacecorps.gov/wws/stories/stories.cfm?psid=981.

"How to Deal with a Bad Gag Reflex." Dental Fear Central. www.dentalfearcentral.org/fears/gagging.

"NOVA Science Now: The Science of Picky Eaters." Video/television/online broadcast. www.pbs.org/wgbh/nova/body/science-picky-eaters.html.

"Roasted Broccoli with Smoked Paprika Vinaigrette and Marcona Almonds," submitted by arielleclementine. www.food52.com/recipes/2625_roasted_broccoli_with_smoked_paprika_vinaigrette_and_marcona_almonds.

"Test Your Tastebuds." www.bbc.co.uk/science/humanbody/body/articles/senses/tongue_experiment.shtml.

"Tips for the Management of the Gagging Patient." Dental Fears Research Clinic, University of Washington. www.dentalfearcentral.org/media/tips_gag_reflex.pdf.

"Tongue Test Identifies Supertasters," March 24, 2003. http://news.bbc.co.uk/2/hi/health/2880471.stm.

ACKNOWLEDGMENTS

They say it takes a village to raise a child. I think it probably takes at least a hamlet and the entire Internet to write a book. I have a lot of people to thank, so bear with me and please stand when you read your name:

Thank-yous go out to the Lady Aye, Dr. Dorothy Burk, Brett and Elan Emerson, Dr. Sarah Nabai, Michael Procopio, Todd Robbins, Karen Ross, Amy Sargent, Gretchen Schuessler, Marianna Thorn, Professor Virginia Utermohlen, and Dr. Nancy Zucker for talking to me and answering my (sometimes bizarre) questions.

To the folks at Monell Chemical Senses Center in Philadelphia, including Amin Khoshnevisan, Johan Lundstrom, Marcia Pelchat, Leslie Stein, and Chuck Wysocki, I appreciate all the time you spent with me. Most of all I am grateful to my DNA Camp counselors at Monell. Thank you, Dani Reed, Antti Knaapila, Anna Lysenko, Sarah Lipchock, and Daniel Hwang for inviting and welcoming me to your lab, where I learned a crapload about taste, smell, genes, and the Ukraine. You tried your hardest, and if I butchered the genotyping process, it's not your fault.

Thank you to all the picky eaters (or picky eater adjacents) who opened up to me: Jeff Alexander, Lora Poppler Alexander, Jon Bourgault, Julie Burba, Chi-An Chien, Doug Cress, Anita Crotty, Craig Demel, Jane Tunks Demel, Jasmine Guillory, Keith Keller, Katie Lambert, Kira, Melissa, Annie Maiser, Anne and Jim McKinney, Joyce Slaton, Susan Tankersley, Jess Thomson,

Sean Timberlake, Molly Watson, and Amy Watts. Finally, thanks to Courtney and Keely Jensen for their feats of bravery as I performed picky eating experiments on them.

This project wouldn't have gone anywhere were it not for my agent and publishing world fairy godmother at Levine Greenberg Literary Agency, Lindsay Edgecombe. She's an indefatigable cheerleader, a patient ego stroker, and a supportive brainstormer. She rocks.

I am indebted to everyone at Perigee Books who put this book together, including publisher John Duff, copyeditor Joan Matthews, publicist Melissa Broder, and Nellys Li for her inspired cover design, but especially to my incredible editor, Jeanette Shaw, for her keen eye and sense of direction, for suffering cheerfully through my bouts of writerly insanity, and for turning me on to *Vampire Diaries*. Without her painstaking and encouraging chapter-by-chapter guidance, this book would be unreadable.

Thank you to Beth Cold, for needles and philosophical discussions. To Catherine Shattuck for her okra and many honest and healing conversations about our struggles with writing. And to Catherine and Jeff Shattuck both for being my marketing gurus. Meredith Arthur for having a very frank discussion about what it would be like to write the book but especially for excitedly supporting me when I went ahead and did it anyway. Meghan Laslosky for her sympathetic support and her brainstorming sessions. Sarah Bunting for giving me my first writing job, making me a better writer, and for being not just an early reader, but also a stalwart friend and a hysterical collaborator.

I am so lucky to be surrounded by an intense battery of friends, online and in person, so my affectionate thanks also go out to Shauna Ahern, Joy Alferness, Carol Blymire, Sam Breach, Jeanne Brophy, Amy Cleary, Heather Cocks, Rachel Cohen,

Nanita Cranford, Anita Crotty, Katie Ginder-Vogel, Gudrun Enger, Genie Gratto, Jennifer Jeffrey, Fatemeh Khatibloo, Kristen LaGrange, Al Lowe, Jen Maiser, Jessica Morgan, Suzanne Randolph, Genevieve Rajewski, Jane Tunks, and Nicole Weaver, all of who called, emailed, or Tweeted their never-ending support during this process.

To my parents, Vern and Gretchen Vander Weide, for firmly believing that everything I wrote was wonderful. Their sometimes misguided literary sense is clearly proof of their love. To my mother-in-law, Judy Lucianovic, for a month of Henry-wrangling and for wanting to ensure that there was going to be enough "Stephanie" in the book. To my older sister and fellow picky eater, Jennie, and to my little sister, Vanessa, for her malaprops and for always having an opinion on what jeans I should be wearing and which shampoo I should be using.

To Mark for believing in me, talking me through my blocks, and for always giving me his share of the fresh coffee and pie. To my Henry, just for being alive.

Finally, to my father-in-law, Bill. I wish you were still with us.